The Causes and Behavioral Consequences of Disasters

Sasha Rudenstine • Sandro Galea

The Causes and Behavioral Consequences of Disasters

Models Informed by the Global Experience 1950–2005

Springer

Sasha Rudenstine
Department of Epidemiology
Mailman School of Public Health
Columbia University
New York, NY 10032-3727, USA
sr2863@columbia.edu

Sandro Galea
Department of Epidemiology
Mailman School of Public Health
Columbia University
New York, NY 10032-3727, USA
sgalea@columbia.edu

ISBN 978-1-4614-0316-6 e-ISBN 978-1-4614-0317-3
DOI 10.1007/978-1-4614-0317-3
Springer New York Dordrecht Heidelberg London

Library of Congress Control Number: 2011934676

Printed on acid-free paper

Springer is part of Springer Science+Business Media (www.springer.com)

Dedicated to my parents, Zina Steinberg and David Rudenstine, and brother, Aaron Rudenstine (SR)

Dedicated to Margaret, Oliver Luke, and Isabel Tess (SG)

Preface

How can communities reduce their vulnerability to disaster? How does population behavior change during disasters and how does this behavior influence public health during and after these events? How would an integrative approach to disaster preparedness that takes into account the causes and behavioral consequences of disasters enhance population health? This book is our attempt to answer these questions.

While we may have little capacity to stop earthquakes or tsunamis, sound infrastructure and effective political organizations before a hazard strikes, and effective leadership and timely dissemination of information after the hazard all can mitigate the adverse population health consequences of these events. Understanding population behavior in the aftermath of potential disasters can also help us intervene to minimize their short- and long-term health consequences.

Informed by a systematic study of a unique representative database of 360 disasters worldwide, spanning 1950–2005, we provide in this book a framework that can help us understand the causes of disasters. We also present a model of population behavior after these events. We intend these two inextricably linked models to be useful guides for public health disaster preparedness and response efforts.

New York, NY — Sasha Rudenstine
New York, NY — Sandro Galea

Acknowledgements

We would like to thank Dr. Craig Hadley. Our early work together, funded by the Robert Wood Johnson Health and Society "Social context and the consequences of disasters: A mixed methods approach to identifying underlying vulnerabilities and capacities" grant laid the foundations for this book. We would also like to thank Dr. Jennifer Ahern who contributed to some of the concepts articulated here.

We are grateful to the many research assistants who contributed to this book: Aditi Sagdeo, Eric Roberts, Ellen Wan, Scot McCususker, Jamie Laudati, Emily Goldmann, Abdulrahman El-Sayed, David Lai, Jenna Johnson, and Shivani Patel. This book would not be possible without them. Kate Scherzo provided important editorial assistance throughout the writing of the book.

Contents

Part I
The Study of Disasters

Chapter 1
Understanding Disasters

The Growing Importance of Disasters Worldwide

The United States (US) changed in the aftermath of the September 11, 2001 terrorist attacks on New York City. Certainly two wars, one in Afghanistan and one in Iraq, would have been unlikely without the preceding terrorist attacks. The state embarked on extensive infrastructural and logistical transformations aimed at preventing future attacks. This effort resulted in massive changes in the federal bureaucracy with the establishment of the Department of Homeland Security, public health campaigns aimed at educating the general public about the potential threat of disasters, and a seemingly constant heightened state of alert intended to keep the US public vigilant and ready for other future calamities.

And yet by August 29, 2005, when Hurricane Katrina hit land on the Mississippi–Louisiana border, it seemed as though all of the preparedness of the previous 4 years was for naught. Responsible for at least 1,604 deaths in its aftermath, Hurricane Katrina was the deadliest hurricane in the US during the last 75 years. Katrina was also the most expensive natural disaster in US history by far, with costs estimated at $100 billion [1]. Substantial parts of New Orleans remained uninhabitable years after Hurricane Katrina and the population in many other parts of southern Louisiana and Mississippi remains to this day a small fraction of what it was before the hurricane. The US public watched agonizing images of residents of New Orleans being stranded on their roofs, of creaking and overburdened shelters themselves threatened by the storm, and of national leaders floundering on the best course of action. This newest disaster caught one of the world's richest countries unprepared, reflecting how little decision makers had indeed learned from the September 11, 2001 terrorist attacks.

While dramatic and headline-grabbing events such as the September 11, 2001 terrorist attacks and Hurricane Katrina focused public attention on disasters, disasters affecting large numbers of people are by no means a novelty. There were 1,500 disaster declarations by the US Federal Emergency Management Agency

S. Rudenstine and S. Galea, *The Causes and Behavioral Consequences of Disasters: Models Informed by the Global Experience* 1950–2005,
DOI 10.1007/978-1-4614-0317-3_1, © Springer Science+Business Media, LLC 2012

between 1967 and 2007 [2]. Between 1974 and 2003 alone, natural disasters killed approximately more than two million people worldwide and affected another 5.1 billion cumulatively [3].

One observation brought home by the events of 2001 and 2005 is that, in many respects, we are increasingly vulnerable to disasters. There are several reasons for this increase in vulnerability. The movement of populations toward geographically vulnerable areas, particularly floodplains, coastal areas, and areas near geologic fault lines, contributes to the greater potential for natural events to affect larger numbers of people [4, 5]. The rapid pace of industrialization has relied on the development of elaborate infrastructure for extraction of raw natural resources and processing plants, accompanied by regular transportation of commercial and waste products, which are often toxic increasing potential for both individual and population level exposure to hazards. The transformation in economic systems has also been driving shifts in population settlement. The world has been rapidly urbanizing. At the end of the nineteenth century less than 3% of the world's population was living in urban environments, while by 2008, for the first time, more people worldwide are estimated to live in urban compared to rural areas [6, 7]. Of the world's 3.3 billion urban dwellers in 2007, 75% are concentrated in only 25 countries [7]. Many of these urban areas are in low-income countries and are characterized by unstable architecture and minimal disaster preparedness [4]. In addition, as our world becomes more interconnected, disasters that occur in areas characterized by war and ethnic conflict produce complex outcomes that affect entire regions [8, 9].

The Academic Study of Disasters

Despite the pervasiveness of disasters and their increasingly pronounced consequences over time, they appear only fleetingly in the public eye. The episodic nature of disasters makes it difficult for them to persist too long in the public mind. Almost inevitably, once a particular disaster passes public attention moves on to the next colorful issue of the day. Those in positions of power – particularly in politics and policy – generally attend to the acute disaster event when they must, as learned through the Hurricane Katrina experience, but pay scant attention to the *potential* for disaster. The public, informed primarily through a commercial mass media that thrives on high profile events, rarely demands more than this.

It is here that academic discourse has played an invaluable role, maintaining and furthering the conversation on disasters *between* events that capture the public's attention. In so doing, this inquiry has developed our understanding of the causes and consequences of disasters.

There is a long and robust history of the study of disasters in the academic literature that varies by discipline and offers complementary understandings of relevant processes and outcomes. Within the natural sciences, including fields such as geology and meteorology, there is a body of work that considers the physical and infrastructural factors that contribute to disasters. This work has led to the establishment of monitoring strategies and technology that are critical, in many countries worldwide, to anticipate or mitigate the consequences of natural disasters. Within the social sciences, particularly within sociology and demography, the study of social systems and their relations to disasters has flourished. In particular, seminal work in the social sciences has placed emphasis on how social systems may generate vulnerability yet simultaneously protect people from the consequences of these events [10–13].

This book fits squarely within these academic traditions and dwells at the intersection of the social and natural sciences. Our motivation here concerns the health of populations. There is a growing body of work in public health and medicine that occupies itself with features of disasters that may influence population health. Most of this literature focuses on individual experience of disasters and how they affect the physical or mental pathology of the individual after these events. This is to some extent in contrast to the sociological or natural science literature that has focused almost exclusively on the physical and social environment that either results in or shapes the consequences of disasters. We aim to combine insights from the natural and social sciences about the study of disasters with the goal of understanding how these events shape and influence public health. Therefore this book is guided by the work of numerous disciplines, aspects of which have been synthesized and reconstructed to enhance the public health perspective on disasters and their consequences.

We see an ever-growing role for population health sciences in the study of disasters. Public attention to these events continues to center around the potential harms of disasters to the general population and such harms range from death to physical and psychological morbidity. It is increasingly understood that while some adverse health consequences of disasters are inevitable, other adverse outcomes can potentially be mitigated through careful pre-event planning and post-event action. Work in the social and natural sciences teaches us that although all disasters are different, there are common characteristics of disasters that can be expected to be associated with positive or negative consequences of an event. It is our goal to build on the social and natural science tradition of inquiry around the causes of disasters and to provide a framework that can be useful in guiding public health preparedness and response efforts.

This book is divided into four sections. Part 1 reviews the definition of disaster and outlines our systematic review of disasters used in this book. Parts 2 and 3 arise from a systematic review of disasters worldwide summarized in Part 1. Part 2 addresses the causes of disasters. Here we argue that features of the social and physical environment, as well as the response to an event, ultimately result in a "disaster" rather than the event itself. In this section, building on a conceptual model that we present in Chap. 3, we discuss the factors that we suggest shape the public health consequences of disasters, including vulnerabilities and capacities, intermittent stressors and intermittent protectors (defined in Chap. 4). Part 3 examines behavioral consequences of disasters. Here, we propose a conceptual model that we hope will further an understanding of population behavior after disasters. This model is motivated by our appreciation that much of what happens *after* a hazard has occurred is key in shaping the health consequences of the event. We propose a five-stage model that outlines patterns of population behavior after such events. In both Parts 2 and 3 of the book, the discussion of each stage of the conceptual framework is followed by a chapter dedicated to a specific disaster (selected from the database described in detail in Chap. 2) to illustrate the applicability of the model to understanding actual real events. Lastly, Part 4 applies both of our models to one disaster, the September 11, 2001 terrorist attacks on the World Trade Center. In addition, we discuss the implications of our proposed models for public health.

Before moving on to the main chapters of this book, we address here one question that we feel is essential to any discussion of disasters – namely what defines a disaster.

What Is a Disaster?

While at face value this seems like a simple question, it is complex enough to have been the subject of many books. In fact several international bodies have adopted definitions of disasters that are in some respects different. Probably the most widely used definition of disaster, adopted by the International Federation of Red Cross and Red Crescent Societies (IFRC) from the Centre for Research on the Epidemiology of Disasters (CRED), considers an event a disaster if it meets one of four criteria: (1) 10 or more persons dead, (2) 100 or more persons affected, (3) declaration of a state of emergency, or (4) call for international assistance [14, 15] (p200). In contrast, the US Federal Emergency Management Agency relies on a range of factors including the destruction or damage to homes and infrastructure and threats to the health and safety of the public to declare a disaster [2]. Although definitions of disasters have historically been built on the study of natural events [9], as the frequency and type of potential causes of disasters increases definitions have relied less and less on an explicit link between the factors that cause disaster events. For example, a typical definition of disasters, from a recent book on the topic, states, "a potentially traumatic event that is collectively experienced, has an acute onset, and is time-delimited; disasters may be attributed to natural, technological, or human causes" [16] (p4).

Relevant to our framework to follow, researchers working on disasters have found it useful to view the event that triggered negative outcomes separately from the negative outcomes themselves. The term "hazard" often refers to the event rather than the consequences. The distinction between disasters and hazards, however, varies and conflicts between authors [17].

For the study of the health consequences of disasters, we think it productive to consider the event itself as a hazard. This is consistent with the work of Pelling [18] who suggests that the hazard is the "potential harm to individuals or human systems" [18] (p5). Turner [19] also suggests that a hazard is "an event *concentrated in time and space* which threatens a society or a relatively self-sufficient subdivision of a society with major unwanted consequences as a result of the collapse of precautions which had hitherto been culturally accepted as adequate" [19] (pp 755–756).

Although much of this work was referring to natural disasters, we consider here hazards as natural, technological, or other human-made events. In turn, it is the interaction of these hazards with natural, physical, environmental, ecological, or social elements that can generate disasters. Disasters are the consequences of the hazard, but clearly not of the singular action of the hazard. Hazards become disasters only in the context of a specific society with particular vulnerabilities and the mere presence of a hazard may make for a disaster in one context and not in another context [20]. It is the focus of Part 2 of this book to identify the factors that, through interplay with hazards, result in disasters.

One more point is worth elaborating on in this regard. The vast majority of hazards responsible for a single disaster are concentrated in time and space. There are, however, hazards that do not meet this criterion or are concentrated only in space, but not time, or vice versa. For example, the ongoing repeat suicide bombings in Israel may be concentrated in space, but are not concentrated in time. Floods may involve vast areas being then concentrated neither in time nor space. Therefore, while for the most part we can consider most hazards as point events, this clearly does not apply to all hazards. This distinction will become important as we proceed with this book since hazards that occur over a prolonged period of time and those that occur within a short time can have different influences, particularly on patterns of population behavior after these events.

To summarize, we do not attempt to newly define disaster in this book. Conceptually, we are in line with the notion that disasters are collectively experienced and should not be defined by a particular cause. In our selection criteria, as we discuss in Chap. 2, we use the IFRC/CRED definition of disasters [14, 15]. The critical distinction between hazard and disaster informs the remainder of this work. Building on work in the natural sciences, we adopt here the term "hazard" to refer to the event that is often called the "disaster" in the popular and scientific literature. Throughout this book, the acute event, or series of acute events – such as a hurricane, an earthquake, a flood, or a terrorist bomb – is referred to as a *hazard*. The term *disaster* refers to the consequences of the hazard, and, particularly to the intersection of the hazard with the underlying vulnerabilities and capacities that shape the health of populations after these events.

How Can the Study of Disasters Inform Public Health?

We intend this book to be helpful to those interested in the health of populations after disasters with two overarching objectives.

First, understanding the *determinants* of disasters and how hazards become disasters can be invaluable in guiding disaster preparedness efforts. As our national awareness of disasters has increased much effort has been invested within the public health community – both the research and clinical communities – in strengthening public health systems that might be frontline disaster response mechanisms. We fear that such efforts are bound to underperform if they focus exclusively on the hazard alone without considering those features of underlying context that may cause disasters when a hazard occurs. An appreciation of the function of local context in shaping the health of populations after these events may guide public health efforts and maximize our efforts to prepare for such hazards. For example, political leadership that is transparent and accountable can be an essential element of an effective disaster response. Recognition of the role of political institutions during disasters begs for a public health strategy for disaster preparedness that can provide effective and consistent leadership and communication during a disaster. Similarly, as we shall discuss in many examples throughout this book, underlying socioeconomic conditions – both at the population and individual levels – are central in shaping disasters when areas are affected by hazards. Disaster preparedness efforts then must consider where and how these underlying vulnerabilities may be an important concern and adapt both available resources and response programs accordingly.

Second, understanding how social circumstance intersects with the occurrence of hazards to produce disasters is essential for effective public health disaster response. The public health response may range from the provision of food after these events to making psychological counseling services available for members of the population who suffer from psychopathology after these events [8]. For example, the presence of religious groups, organizations, and/or other forms of social cohesion may help provide emotional as well as material support during a disaster. Acknowledgement of the role of these nongovernmental organizations is critical in any planned disaster response strategy. Similarly, structural factors not directly related to disaster management should fall within the domain of public health responses to disasters. Recognizing that areas with different infrastructural development (including architecture as well as publicly administered water and sanitation resources) will have very different capacities to respond to a hazard is essential in thinking about potential disaster response.

References

1. Department of Homeland Security. The First Year After Hurricane Katrina: What the Federal Government Did. http://www.dhs.gov/katrina. Accessed 10 Oct 2008.
2. Federal Emergency Management Agency. http://www.fema.gov/hazard/index.shtm. Accessed 10 Oct 2008.
3. Guha-Sapir D, Hargitt D, Hoyois P. Thirty years of natural disasters 1974–2003: the numbers. Louvain-la-Neuve, Belgium: Centre for Research on the Epidemiology of Disasters; 2004.
4. Sapir DG, Lechat MF. Reducing the impact of natural disasters: Why aren't we better prepared? Health Pol Plan. 1986;1:118–26.
5. McGranahan G, Balk D, Anderson B. The rising tide: assessing the risks of climate change and human settlements in low elevation coastal zones. Environ Urban. 2007;19:17–37.
6. Clark D. Urban World/Global City. London: Routledge; 2003.
7. World Urbanization Prospects. World Urbanization Prospects: the 2007 revision. New York: United Nations; 2008.
8. Noji EK. The public health consequences of disasters. New York: Oxford University Press; 1997.

9. Waeckerle JF, Lillibridge SR, Burkle Jr FM, Noji EK. Disaster medicine: challenges for today. Ann Emerg Med. 1994;23:715–8.
10. Quarantelli EL. Disaster studies: An historical analysis of the influence of basic sociology and applied use on the research done in the last 35 years. DRC Preliminary Paper 111. Symposium on social structure and disaster: conception and measurement. College of William and Mary, Williamsburg, VA; 1986.
11. Sen A. Food, economics and entitlements. In: Dreze J, Sen A, editors. The political economy of hunger. Oxford, UK: Clarendon; 1990. p. 50–67.
12. Bohle HG, Downing TE, Watts MJ. Climate change and social vulnerability: toward a sociology and geography of food insecurity. Glob Environ Change. 1994;4:37–48.
13. Oliver-Smith A. Disaster context and causation: an overview of changing perspectives in disaster research. In: Oliver-Smith A, editor. Natural disasters and cultural responses. Williamsburg, VA: College of William & Mary; 1986.
14. Centre for Research on the Epidemiology of Disasters. Emergency Events Database. http://www.emdat.be/. Accessed 8 Apr 2009.
15. International Federation of Red Cross and Red Crescent Societies (IFRC). World disasters report: focus on neglected crises. 2006.
16. Norris FH. Methods for disaster mental health research. New York: The Guilford Press; 2006.
17. Alexander D. Natural disasters. London: UCL Press; 1993.
18. Pelling M. The vulnerability of cities: natural disasters and social resilience. Sterling, VA: Earthscan Publications; 2003.
19. Turner BA. The development of disasters: a sequence model for the analysis of the origin of disasters. Sociol Rev. 1976;24:753–74.
20. Bankoff G, Frerks G, Hilhorst D. Mapping vulnerability: disasters, development, and people. London: Earthscan Publications; 2004.

Chapter 2
Broadening Our Conception of Disasters and Their Consequences

The comprehensive study of disasters requires a multidisciplinary perspective. While both the methods and the object of inquiry may have disciplinary overlap, relevant expertise and uses of these methods vary across disciplines. In this chapter we first discuss the disciplinary perspectives that guide this work and on which we build our inference. Second, we introduce and summarize the dataset that was collected and analyzed, forming the backbone of this book.

The Study of Disasters Is Multidisciplinary

Perspectives from several disciplines, including cultural anthropology, sociology, psychology, epidemiology, architecture, engineering, and risk assessment, inform this book. We build on insights from cultural anthropology that has effectively used ethnography as a method to understand human societies and individuals embedded within them. In-depth interviews and participant observation have proven to be useful ethnographic tools to understand the individual experience of a disaster and the role of culture in shaping that experience. Sociology has long aimed to understand the experience and different reactions of groups affected by disasters. For example, after a fire at the Hamilton Distributing Company and Ephrata Paint Store in Ephrata, Pennsylvania, Fischer et al. [1] studied evacuation behavior of residents living near the hazard. The study found that evacuation behavior was linked to the type of information (i.e., clarity and frequency of message, and source of information) and the composition of household members at risk (i.e., presence of children) [1, 2].

We also draw on insight from several health disciplines that have studied the physical and mental health consequences of these events. Psychology uses diagnostic interviews to assess the mental health consequences of disasters, particularly among those who are immediate victims to or participants in some aspects of the pre- or post-disaster process. For example, after the World Trade Center disaster in

S. Rudenstine and S. Galea, *The Causes and Behavioral Consequences of Disasters: Models Informed by the Global Experience* 1950–2005,
DOI 10.1007/978-1-4614-0317-3_2, © Springer Science+Business Media, LLC 2012

New York City in 2001, Gross [3] measured posttraumatic stress disorder and other psychological consequences among World Trade Center clean-up and recovery workers. This research demonstrates the existence of far-reaching health effects of disasters and helps to identify population needs after a disaster. Epidemiologists have employed quantitative studies to measure the consequences of disasters on a defined population that may or may not have been directly affected by the immediate disaster. These studies survey a community at either a single time point or over time. As an example of cross-sectional studies, epidemiologists have identified the prevalence of major depression and posttraumatic stress disorder among the general population after the Madrid train bombings on March 11, 2004 [4]. Longitudinal data, such as a four-wave panel study of families affected by major flooding and mudslides in Mexico in 1999, offer a glimpse at long-term consequences of disasters and patterns of recovery [5].

We are also informed by the emphasis on technical approaches and structural features that are the hallmark of other fields of practice and research concerned with disasters. Engineering, for example, uses surveying of physical structures to assess the degree of architectural stability of buildings and the extent to which structures are vulnerable to the effects of disasters. Architects have studied the design flaws and functionality that may permit a hazard to progress to a disaster. Ultimately, we also build on insights from the field of risk assessment, which has traditionally provided theories of probabilities of hazards and loss. For example, Yue et al. [6] have created models to determine where and at what intensity Aeolian sand disasters will occur in northern China. Risk assessment has been invaluable to our understanding of "what hazard events may occur," "what is the probability of each event," and finally, "what is the likely loss created by each event" [7, p. 59].

An Empirical Dataset to Extend the Contextual Study of Disasters

Building on, and borrowing from, these diverse disciplinary perspectives, we aimed to extend how we think about disasters and their consequences through an empirical approach, founded on a database that spans time and place. We are motivated by the observation that much of the disaster research to date has focused either on specific disaster outcomes (such as mental health or economic damage) or on how to conceptualize the factors that affect the severity of common disaster types (such as, for example, architectural enquiry into how buildings may withstand earthquakes). Our intent then was to adopt and borrow from many of the aforementioned disciplinary approaches and their underlying theoretical frameworks to ask ourselves how we can better understand the factors that drive population health after a disaster. First, we set out to identify the vulnerabilities and capacities that may intersect with a hazard to produce health outcomes after disasters, and describe how these vulnerabilities and capacities interact with stressors and protectors. Second we identify a model of population behavior after these events.

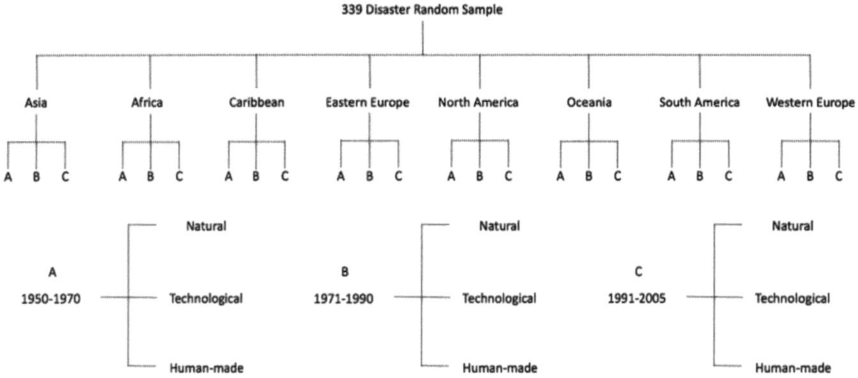

Diagram 2.1 Random sample of disasters comprised of 72 unique combinations of disaster type, time period, and place

Central to our work is an empirical dataset of 339 disasters, which cover different types of disasters over time and place. We constructed our database from a comprehensive list of disasters that took place between 1950 and 2005 and that met at least one of the four criteria for a disaster, as defined by the Centre for Research on the Epidemiology of Disasters (CRED) and the IFRC: [8, 9] (1) at least 10 killed, (2) at least 100 affected, (3) declaration of a state of emergency, or (4) appeal for international assistance. Three primary categories of disasters were considered: natural, technological, and human-made. Natural and technological disasters were sampled from comprehensive lists of disasters globally compiled by the CRED [8]. In an effort to compile an exhaustive human-made disaster list, we used comprehensive lists of all terrorist (broadly defined) attacks created by the Memorial Institute for the Prevention of Terrorism (MIPT) [10]. The MIPT's lists integrate information from the RAND Terrorism Chronology and RAND-MIPT Terrorism incident Databases, the Terrorism Indictment Database, and DFI International's Research on Terrorist Organizations. We cross-checked the MIPT lists with several other databases to ensure that a comprehensive list of terrorist attacks was included. Finally, we compiled several databases of the human-made disasters that do not fall under the terrorism category (e.g., wars and ethnic conflict) to create the final pool of disasters for this category [11, 12].

Using this comprehensive sampling frame, we randomly selected a subset of disasters for each category (natural, technological, and human-made) for each of two strata, time period and geographic region. We stratified disasters into three time periods – 1950–1970, 1971–1990, and 1991–2005. Eight geographic regions were identified: North America (the USA and Canada), South and Central America (including Mexico), Caribbean (including Puerto Rico), Africa, Western Europe, Asia, Eastern Europe (including Russia), and Oceania. Thus, 72 unique combinations of disaster type, time period, and place were generated. A total of five disasters were selected for each of these 72 combinations to create the final dataset that could include 360 disasters. There were fewer than five disasters in some of the cells, hence the final total of disasters reviewed was 339 (Diagram 2.1, Table 2.1).

Table 2.1 Distribution of disasters by disaster type, time period, place

	Asia	Africa	Caribbean	Eastern Europe	North America	Oceania	South America	Western Europe
1950–1970								
Natural	5	5	5	5	5	5	5	5
Technological	5	5	3	5	5	1	5	5
Human-made	5	5	5	5	5	1	5	5
1971–1990								
Natural	5	5	5	5	5	5	5	5
Technological	5	5	5	5	5	5	5	5
Human-made	5	5	5	5	5	2	5	5
1991–2005								
Natural	5	5	5	5	5	5	5	5
Technological	5	5	5	5	5	5	5	5
Human-made	5	5	2	5	5	0	5	5
Total	45	45	40	45	45	29	45	45

For each of the disasters, we collected information on the characteristics of the instigating hazard, such as type of hazard, magnitude, and duration. We traced the local and international response to the disaster by examining records of material and economic assistance, rescue workers, medical aid (including supplies, medicines, health care professionals, and refugee camps), and government and NGO actions. We also conducted an extensive review of relevant academic research studies, governmental reports, and nonprofit emergency response organizations (e.g., Red Cross) reports to obtain information on the short- and long-term outcomes of the disaster, including economic damage as well as injury, mortality, disease, displacement, mental health effects, and other related factors. We turned to qualitative sources (personal accounts, media reports, and government reports) to better capture the individual, local, national, and international reaction, response, and recovery from the disaster.

In addition to the disaster and its aftermath, we gathered information on the regional and local context. Statistical data at the national and regional level, including demographic information such as urban versus rural distribution, population density, literacy, and linguistic groups in the region, were compiled, along with economic, political, and historical characteristics of the region. Our objective was to synthesize descriptive historical and current information for the affected region to best understand the political, economic, and social institutions governing the affected population contemporaneous with the disaster.

Our Contribution to the Study of Disasters

Using our multidisciplinary perspective and empirical dataset, we aim to contribute to, as well as further, the current discussion on etiology and consequences of disasters. In Part 2, we explore the influence of various contextual factors – which, as later discussed, we consider to be classified as vulnerabilities, capacities, intermittent stressors, or intermittent protectors – on hazards and how they intersect to produce particular disasters. In Part 3, we begin a dialog about population behaviors after a disaster by articulating stages of such behavior. In this discussion we take into account the influence of underlying vulnerabilities and capacities as well as global variation driven by cross-national contextual differences that extend beyond these categories.

References

1. Fischer HW, Stine GF, Stoker BL, Trowbridge ML, Drain EM. Evacuation behavior: why do some evacuate while others do not? A case study of the Ephrata, Pennsylvania (USA) evacuation. Disaster Prev Manag. 1995;4:30–6.
2. Fischer HW. Response to disaster: fact versus fiction and its perpetuation. The sociology of disaster. 2nd ed. New York: University of America, Inc.; 1998.
3. Gross R, Neria Y, Tao XG, Massa J, Ashwell L, Davis K, et al. Posttraumatic stress disorder and other psychological sequelae among World Trade Center clean up and recovery workers. Ann N Y Acad Sci. 2006;1071:495–9.
4. Miguel-Tobal JJ, Cano-Vindel A, Gonzalez-Ordi H, et al. PTSD and depression after the Madrid March 11 train bombings. J Trauma Stress. 2006;19:69–80.
5. Norris FH, Murphy AD, Baker CK, Perilla JL. Postdisaster PTSD over four waves of a panel study of Mexico's 1999 flood. J Trauma Stress. 2004;17:283–92.
6. Yue Y, Wang J, Zou X, Shi P. Risk assessment of Aeolian sand disaster on city in sandy area of northern china based on RS, GIS and models. J Nat Disasters. 2008;17:15–20.
7. Smith K. Environmental hazards: assessing risk and reducing disaster. 3rd ed. London: Routledge; 2001.
8. Centre for Research on the Epidemiology of Disasters. Emergency events database. http://www.emdat.be/. Accessed 8 Apr 2009.
9. International Federation of Red Cross and Red Crescent Societies (IFRC). World disasters report: focus on neglected crises. Geneva: IFRC; 2006.
10. Memorial Institute for the Prevention of Terrorism (MIPT). Terrorism incidents and significant dates. http://www.terrorisminfo.mipt.org/incidentcalendar.asp. Accessed 8 Apr 2009.
11. OnWar. Wars of the world. http://www.onwar.com/aced/index.htm. Accessed 8 Apr 2009.
12. Timelines.Info. Conflict and war. http://www.timelines.info/. Accessed 8 Apr 2009.

Part II
Causes of Disasters

Chapter 3
The Missing Role of Context: A Conceptual Model

All hazards do not end in disaster. From a public health perspective we are primarily concerned with preempting adverse health outcomes caused by hazards, particularly at the population level. To that end, it is apposite that both the tradition of disaster research and epidemiology are particularly occupied with identifying the population at risk of experiencing a disaster. The notion of vulnerabilities and capacities has been discussed in a variety of disciplines to describe characteristics of individuals, societies, and environments in relation to external threats to a population. Vulnerabilities are understood to enable negative outcomes, while capacities enable positive outcomes. This chapter will focus on the conceptualization of disaster risk, as defined in much of the academic literature, as vulnerabilities and capacities. Our models, presented in this book, pay special attention to the interaction between vulnerabilities and capacities, with each other and with the hazard, to ultimately produce or avert a disaster.

Understanding the Causes and Consequences of Disasters

We propose here a conceptual model that specifies the interrelations among the key determinants of the consequences of hazards, i.e., disasters; this model guides our work. The remainder of the book will focus on illustrating the applicability of the model using case studies from the empirical disaster dataset described in Chap. 2. In this chapter we introduce the model and in subsequent chapters we elaborate on its constituent elements. We present the overall model first as a means of orienting the reader and of organizing the content to come. This model emerges from the discussion to follow about the nature of each of these dimensions and from the in-depth case studies that are interspersed with the content chapters.

Several disciplines have come to agree that the initial hazard, whether it be natural, technological, or human-made, is not an isolated predictor of the events or outcomes to follow. Rather, preexisting characteristics of the affected region intersect

S. Rudenstine and S. Galea, *The Causes and Behavioral Consequences of Disasters: Models Informed by the Global Experience* 1950–2005,
DOI 10.1007/978-1-4614-0317-3_3, © Springer Science+Business Media, LLC 2012

with the hazard to shape the magnitude of the consequences of the hazard [1–3]. These preexisting characteristics can produce adverse consequences [4–6] but can also mitigate the consequences of hazards [3, 7–10]. We use here the term "vulnerabilities" for the former, and "capacities" for the latter. While much of the research in the area has focused on how specific features of context are "vulnerabilities," recent work has also drawn our attention to the unique role of "capacities" [3, 7, 8]. In some respects capacities are the "flip side" of vulnerabilities, and therefore the absence of a vulnerability is a capacity. As we shall discuss, however, we think that there is merit to considering vulnerabilities and capacities jointly, highlighting not only the unique contributions of factors that may serve one or another function, but also the observation that some factors may typically function as vulnerabilities, while others may typically function as capacities. We further develop our conceptual framework by introducing the notion of intermittent protectors and intermittent stressors. We consider these to be transient factors that intersect with underlying vulnerabilities and capacities to shape the consequences of hazards.

Our model of disaster development therefore consists of three stages. First, the context in which a disaster strikes is characterized by vulnerabilities and capacities. Features of the underlying context rest on a vulnerability–capacity continuum and their role as vulnerabilities or capacities depends on their influence in exacerbating, or protecting against, the adverse consequences of hazards that affect regions and populations. Second, a hazard occurs that intersects with existing vulnerabilities and capacities, defining the severity of the disaster. Temporally the vulnerabilities and capacities predate the hazard, although, in the case of chronic hazards, the hazards themselves may shape the underlying vulnerabilities and capacities. Third, intermittent stressors and intermittent protectors act coincident with, or soon after, the hazard. They become apparent only after the hazard initiates, and have the potential to enhance or mitigate the severity of disaster outcomes. The figure represents this model pictorially.

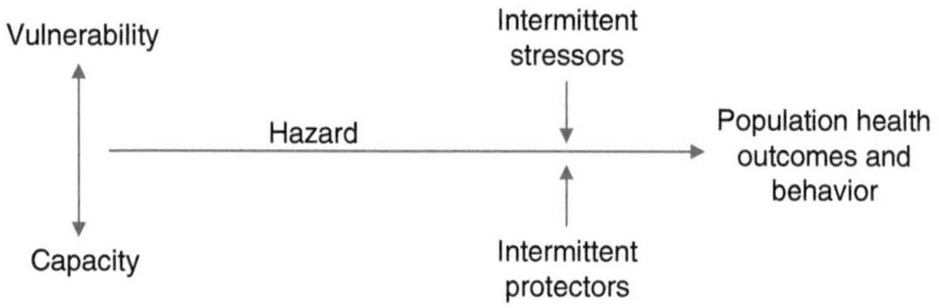

Before discussing each of the elements of this conceptual model in more detail, we present here one example of a hazard – a cholera outbreak – and its consequences, as shaped by vulnerabilities, capacities, and intermittent stressors and protectors.

From late 1997 through much of 1998 Uganda suffered from a fast spreading and lethal cholera outbreak, its first in 25 years [11]. Over the course of approximately 10 months, more than 26 of Uganda's 45 districts were affected; out of approximately

43,911 cases, 1,777 persons are reported to have died [12, 13]. Intense rains and subsequent flooding in Eastern Uganda precipitated the outbreak; contaminated water supplies and elevated degrees of poor hygiene were the outcome of the country's inadequate infrastructure for draining floodwaters [14, 15]. Uganda's conditions were ripe for an epidemic [16].

As the flood levels rose in Eastern Uganda, several factors interacted to influence the spread of cholera throughout the country. Many neighborhoods had neither latrines nor toilets, and poor hygiene contributed to the epidemic developing and spreading readily to nearby communities [17]. In addition, the country lacked sufficient funding or medically trained professionals to quickly address the medical needs of those affected [15]. On the other hand, prior to the outbreak, Uganda had an established branch of the Red Cross, which was critical in slowing the spread of the epidemic. The organization, which was staffed and well structured, was capable of efficiently deploying over 100 volunteers who flocked to the central offices in the wake of the floods and epidemic [18]. Government officials and the country's health ministry launched countrywide surveillance of the outbreak and opened Cholera Treatment Centers in those regions most severely affected by the epidemic. Both of these efforts allowed the government to effectively allocate its few resources, medical supplies, and personnel to those regions most affected by the outbreak, as measured by the number of cases present and the speed of transmission [15].

As the epidemic spread throughout the country several unexpected factors hindered the country's efforts to mitigate the consequences of the outbreak. The flooding easily destroyed existing latrines throughout the country because of their minimal structural supports. The result was vast contamination of water supplies and greater spread of Cholera [17]. Further, flooding wiped out roads, slowing response efforts throughout the country [11]. District medical teams and health officials closed schools, eating houses, and lodges and registered all the homes without latrines with the government throughout the country in an effort to reduce the spread of cholera in densely populated public locales [19].

Ten months after the cholera outbreak began reports noted a slowing of new cases throughout the country. Although the overall governmental effort was successful at controlling the outbreak, the underlying vulnerabilities (i.e., poor hygiene) and intermittent stressors (i.e., contamination of water supplies) substantially influenced the scope of the epidemic that followed the cholera outbreak.

Therefore, our overall model builds on prominent explanations of disaster etiology in the scientific literature and extends these explanations in two significant ways. First, we consider preexisting characteristics along a continuum, suggesting that key underlying features of context can contribute to the exacerbation, or mitigation, of the consequences of a hazard depending on an interaction with other conditions in a particular time and place. Secondly, we acknowledge that there are neutral preexisting characteristics that will act as a vulnerability or capacity *only* in the presence of an external stressor (the hazard). We term these characteristics intermittent stressors and intermittent protectors, respectively. In subsequent chapters, we will elaborate on each of these elements and illustrate their operation with specific disaster case studies.

References

1. Cardona O. The need for rethinking the concepts of vulnerability and risk from a holistic perspective: A necessary review and criticism for effective risk management. In: Bankoff G, Frerks G, Hilhorst D, editors. Mapping vulnerability: disasters, development and people. Sterling, VA: Earthscan; 2004. p. 10.
2. Hilhorst D. Complexity and diversity: Unlocking social domains of disaster response. In: Bankoff G, Frerks G, Hilhorst D, editors. Mapping vulnerability: disasters, development and people. Sterling, VA: Earthscan; 2004. p. 52.
3. Wisner B, Blaikie PM, Cannon T, Davis I. At risk: natural hazards, people's vulnerability and disasters. 2nd ed. New York, NY: Routledge; 2005.
4. Lewis J. Development in disaster-prone places: studies of vulnerability. London: Intermediate Technology; 1999.
5. Wisner B, Luce HR. Disaster vulnerability: scale, power and daily life. Geo J. 1993;30:127–40.
6. Eakin H, Luers AL. Assessing the vulnerability of social-environmental systems. Annu Rev Environ Resour. 2006;31:365.
7. Wisner B. Assessment of capability and vulnerability. In: Bankoff G, Frerks G, Hilhorst D, editors. Mapping vulnerability: disasters, development and people. Sterling, VA: Earthscan; 2004. p. 183.
8. Davis I. Progress in analysis of social vulnerability and capacity. In: Bankoff G, Frerks G, Hilhorst D, editors. Mapping vulnerability: disasters, development and people. London: Earthscan; 2004. p. 128.
9. Anderson MB, Woodrow PJ. Rising from the ashes: development strategies in times of disaster. Boulder, CO: Lynne Rienner Publishers; 1998.
10. Anderson MB. You save my life today, but for what tomorrow?: Some moral dilemmas of humanitarian aid. In: Moore J, editor. Hard choices: moral dilemmas in humanitarian intervention. New York: Rowman and Littlefield Publishers; 1998. p. 137–56.
11. Cholera spreads in East Africa as rain cuts vital link. Agence France-Presse. December 20, 1997.
12. World Health Organization. Cholera in Uganda, update. *Africa News*. September 21, 1998.
13. Malaria kills 328 in Southwestern Uganda. Xinhua News Agency. February 8, 1998.
14. Cholera claims 77 in Uganda. Xinhua News Agency. December 20, 1997.
15. Uganda establishes Cholera control centers. Xinhua News Agency. January 1, 1998.
16. International Federation of Red Cross and Red Crescent Societies. Eastern Africa: Post-Flood Rehabilitation and Food Security. http://www.reliefweb.int/rw/rwb.nsf/db900sid/OCHA-64DBP3?OpenDocument. Accessed 7 July 2009.
17. Cholera kills 9 in E. Uganda. Xinhua News Agency. December 7, 1997.
18. Cholera claims 188 Ugandans in three weeks. Xinhua News Agency. December 30, 1997.
19. Etengu N. Cholera death toll at 236. New Vision. December 31, 1997.

Chapter 4
The Continuum of Vulnerabilities and Capacities

The role of local context is paramount in determining both the nature of the disaster that may arise from a hazard and whether a pre-existing characteristic will indeed become a vulnerability or a capacity. A vulnerability in a particular setting may be neutral or even a capacity at another time, place, or when confronting a different hazard. Vulnerabilities and capacities may include, among others, features of political governance, demography, culture, economy, history, geography, and physical environment. A vulnerability-capacity continuum casts in bold relief the centrality of the pre-disaster context and the complexity of forces that may counteract, amplify, or co-exist with one another. For example, geographic isolation may protect against external conquest and may be responsible for a locally strong political system, which in turn might protect a population affected by a hazard. On the other hand, geographic isolation can also reduce the availability of outside aid when needed. A weak economy may limit the resources available to attend to the hazard, creating a disaster. Conversely, a strong economy characterized by substantial socioeconomic disparities can exacerbate the influence of a hazard, particularly among marginalized groups. Strong community organizations may serve as a mechanism for support in the aftermath of a disaster. Here, we discuss the ways in which particular vulnerabilities and capacities may influence hazards to produce disasters.

History

The history of a region and of a community substantially shapes vulnerabilities and capacities. Events of the past, which have shaped the current context of a community in innumerable ways, interact with hazards to potentially produce or reduce risk of disaster [1]. Historically determined vulnerabilities include, for example, settlement patterns (coastal), social composition (diversity or marginalization), and the present system of governance [1].

S. Rudenstine and S. Galea, *The Causes and Behavioral Consequences of Disasters: Models Informed by the Global Experience* 1950–2005,
DOI 10.1007/978-1-4614-0317-3_4,

For example, colonial history may shape cultural preferences that affect disaster risk. An example is the Peru Earthquake of 1950. Oliver-Smith suggests that prior to the colonization of Peru by Spaniards, Inca populations did not experience significant mortality or destruction from the geological hazard of earthquakes [2]. He attributes this to the ability of communities to develop building infrastructure and urban design that were well adapted to local conditions and sufficiently malleable to deal with new conditions and hazards. The adaptive insight that informed traditional Incan architecture was disrupted by colonization and replaced with architectural tastes unsuitable for the region. In effect, the inappropriate architecture that rendered Peru susceptible to devastating effects of earthquakes was a byproduct of the nation's colonial history.

Political and organizational history may be an important determinant of emergency aid after a disaster [3]. Colonization, in particular a history of government partiality along social, ethnic, and economic lines, may trigger ethnic conflict and revolts in a population. Papua New Guinea suffered a decade long conflict between government officials supporting a powerful and wealthy Australian mining company and natives who lost land and rivers to the mine [4].

Geography

In understanding disasters, place matters. Geography is related to climate, which in turn affects both the nature of the hazard as well as the possibility of developing measures to counteract hazards. Human settlement has been determined by the availability of water and land resources and/or by land availability, which historically hinges on geography. Settling alongside water sources may have been crucial for survival, but puts a community at greater risk for flooding. Many of the staple grains consumed throughout the world today are more fertile on level lowlands where rainfed agriculture can thrive; however these are also the regions more prone to flooding. Following a flood in much of Columbia in 2005, landslides and flooding destroyed significantly more homes near rivers and mountains than those which were situated in less vulnerable environments [5].

The potential to develop capacities against hazards is also influenced by climate, and thus geography. For example, the quality of physical infrastructure will often reflect a combination of both climate and resources. Roads are an excellent example. In the Midwest United States, deicing chemicals used to keep highways drivable in the winter (including salt) will cause accelerated deterioration of the concrete. In regions with monsoon rains, heavy and concentrated rainfall can cause severe erosion and therefore completely compromise roads and oftentimes bridges. The existence and maintenance of road infrastructure is critical for disaster response. Iran struggled to meet the needs of those affected after an earthquake in 1956 due to the lack of roads throughout the country [6].

Demography

Population characteristics interact with the hazard and other existing vulnerabilities and capacities to shape disasters. Population size relative to the area of political boundaries and institutional capacities of a region may create a situation in which even a modest hazard can become disastrous. If many people are affected in a smaller region of a larger political state, management of the hazard ostensibly will be easier. On the other hand, if only a few people are affected, but this encompasses a greater fraction of the population and they are spread over wider administrative boundaries, then it may become a bigger problem for institutions to provide necessary support.

The age distribution of the population also influences the eventual disaster. The young and old tend to be disproportionately affected by hazards. These cohorts may be more vulnerable to particular types of hazards, such as infectious diseases, and generally have less control over resources. Countries with higher fertility and a younger population experience greater mortality during disasters and this is particularly apparent during complex emergencies that challenge food security [7]. Similarly, there is a growing elderly population in many wealthier countries that may present a different kind of population vulnerability. The economic base for hazard management and disaster recovery may also fall short of needs if the burden of productivity is falling on the shoulders of a smaller fraction of the total population. However, population distribution and disaster risk are both dynamic. A younger population will grow into a large, and possibly productive, labor force. An elderly population represents an important capacity with respect to social cohesiveness and traditional knowledge [8].

Culture

Cultural norms may operate in complex ways, affect disaster formation and mitigation, and act alongside political and economic factors to particularly influence individual and group response to hazards. Social cohesion and stability may minimize chronic stress and therefore be important in averting such events. Social factors may also be important in mitigating or containing the disaster. Volunteerism and civilian cooperation may act in concert with political institutions charged with returning an affected area to normalcy. It may also be the case that lack of functioning public institutions may create a need for greater cooperation among the private/individual sector and may be a very important force in rehabilitating an affected group. Many forms of response services and efforts were visible following the Lockerbie plane crash of Pan Am Flight 103 in 1988. Civilians were an essential support structure for recovery efforts, helping, for example, distribute food and drink to rescue workers. Different local agencies provided instrumental support by providing social supports for the families of those who had died in the crash [9]. Finally, economic stability of the country and the influx of donations following the crash provided a secure foundation for local institutions to flourish as a caretaking community.

Political Factors

Political will to act after a hazard strikes is a critical determining factor in the acute development of a disaster. Political institutions are specifically charged with maintaining the safety of the public and therefore are recognized as having crucial responsibilities throughout the disaster and its aftermath. Horrendous prison conditions were just one factor leading to the devastating outcome of a prison fire in Caracas, Venezuela in 1996. Political decisions to forfeit the safety of inmates resulted in over-occupation of the prison by approximately 700 inmates (maximum capacity was reported at 1,000, at the time of the fire 1,700 inmates were being housed at the prison). In addition, after the fire broke out sufficient efforts were not made to put it out leading to over 24 men dying in the flames [10, 11].

Economic Factors

Economic systems, like cultural and historical factors, are generally considered to have only a distal influence on the disaster. They are, however, crucial to the chronic forces that drive vulnerability to disasters and the development of capacities against them. Poverty at the individual and institutional level may play a central role in determining susceptibility to disaster, while wealth tends to make both individuals and institutions more resilient to them. After a dam collapse in the Mendoza of Argentina in 1970, floodwaters swept through the city killing 25 and sweeping away anything in its path. Thousands were left homeless. Most were residents of slum dwellings whose homes were not as structurally sound as those of the more wealthy residents of the city whose homes withstood the effects of the flooding [12].

Physical Environment

A particular factor may be a vulnerability in one setting and a capacity in another. Consider the course of two different hazards influenced by the same structural feature. A drought occurred in Papua New Guinea in 1997 because of an El Nino event (a modifying factor). Due to poor transportation infrastructure in Papua New Guinea, the governing provinces were unable to transport materials and substantive supplies to many of the regions affected by the drought. This is a familiar story in many parts of the world. Conversely, adequate transportation infrastructure can be an important capacity in areas exposed to strong hazards. A fire broke out at Hartford Hospital, Connecticut, US on December 8, 1961. Patients were immediately transferred in ambulances to nearby hospitals, allowing them to escape from injury due to the fire itself and to receive continued care for the conditions for which they were admitted in the first place. While transportation of food relief was limited by road infrastructure threatening the food security of hundreds of thousands of people in Papua New Guinea, the high quality roads and vehicles in the west saved hundreds of lives in Connecticut over three decades before.

It is worth noting that these categories of vulnerabilities and capacities may also act as hazards themselves. Destructive fires may be caused by arid conditions in forests or by social tensions turning violent. Earthquakes and riots both cause property destruction and loss of life. Economic recession or floods may be the agent of food scarcity. Again this highlights the contextual nature of disasters; a hazard in one context may play the role of vulnerability in another.

References

1. Kreps GA, Bosworth SL. Disaster, organizing, and role enactment: a structural approach. Am J Sociol. 1993;99:428–63.
2. Oliver-Smith A. Peru's five hundred year earthquake: vulnerability in historical context. In: Oliver-Smith A, Hoffman SM, editors. The angry earth. New York: Routledge; 1999. p. 74–88.
3. Olsen GR, Carstensen N, Høyen K. Humanitarian crises: what determines the level of emergency assistance? Media coverage, donor interests and the aid business. Disasters. 2003; 27:109–26.
4. Chappell T. Doing it tough/PGN leaders warn of hard times ahead. Daily Telegraph. Sep 16, 1998.
5. In Colombia 16 dead, 30 injured in torrential rains. Agence France-Presse. May 7, 2005.
6. Tremors rock quake ridden area in Iran. Chicago Daily Tribune, C 6. Nov 12, 1956.
7. Ezra M, Kiros GE. Household vulnerability to food crisis and mortality in the drought-prone areas of Northern Ethiopia. J Biosoc Sci. 2000;32:395.
8. Wisner B, Blaikie PM, Cannon T, Davis I. At risk: natural hazards, people's vulnerability and disasters. 2nd ed. New York, NY: Routledge; 2005.
9. Gill K, Faux R. Shattered town yearns for a sense of normality. The Times, Issue 63273. Dec 24, 1988.
10. Sequera V. AP photos CAR102105. Associated Press Worldstream (International News). Oct 22, 1996.
11. Venezuela inmates go on hunger strike. United Press International. Oct 28, 1996.
12. Argentine city digs out after 25 die in flood. New York Times, Front 2. Jan 7, 1970.

Chapter 5
Vulnerabilities and Capacities: Venezuela Floods and Mudslides – December 14–16, 1999

In 1999, heavy rainfall in Venezuela [1] triggered mudslides that buried entire villages and cities. The rain lasted 2 weeks [2–4]. In just 2 days, from December 14–16, about 30,000 people were killed. Another 600,000 felt the effects of the mud and water, including thousands who lost their homes [5, 6]. Heavy rainfall and flooding are not uncommon in the area [4], but the mayor of Caracas, Antonio Ledezma, and other officials described the rain as the heaviest in 60 years [1] and the flooding that followed as the country's worst disaster since an earthquake more than 30 years before, in 1967 [7].

Poor districts were the hardest hit, as the rain relentlessly poured into rivers, causing them "to overflow their banks, sweeping through poor districts…(T)he streets were turned into fields of thick mud, strewn with tree trunks, rocks, and boulders" [2]. Nearly one-third of Venezuela's 23 states (Zulia, Falcon, Yaracuy, Nueva Esparta, Carabobo, Tachira, and Miranda), the State of Vargas, and the Federal District of Caracas sustained the most damaging effects [8]. On December 16, 1999, the federal government declared a state of emergency and got to work orchestrating both national and international relief efforts [1, 8].

Numerous people were stranded in marginalized communities, and the weather continued to work against them for several days after the mudslides. Rescue efforts were hindered most in those areas, although rescue workers encountered problems virtually everywhere [9].

The weather finally began to clear on December 19, 3 days after the mudslides ended. Only then, as rescuers gained access to the hardest-hit areas, did the "massive scale of the disaster" become clear [9]. Reporters who made their way to the vicinity discovered "scenes of urbanized canyons, riverside neighborhoods and coastal plains turned into raging torrents with collapsed houses, apartment buildings buried in mud up to the third floor, cars smashed and tossed like discarded aluminum cans" [7]. Thousands of people, "their clothes torn and muddied, their few possessions packed in plastic bags," [10] evacuated their homes in search of food and shelter [11] (Image 5.1).

S. Rudenstine and S. Galea, *The Causes and Behavioral Consequences of Disasters: Models Informed by the Global Experience* 1950–2005,
DOI 10.1007/978-1-4614-0317-3_5,

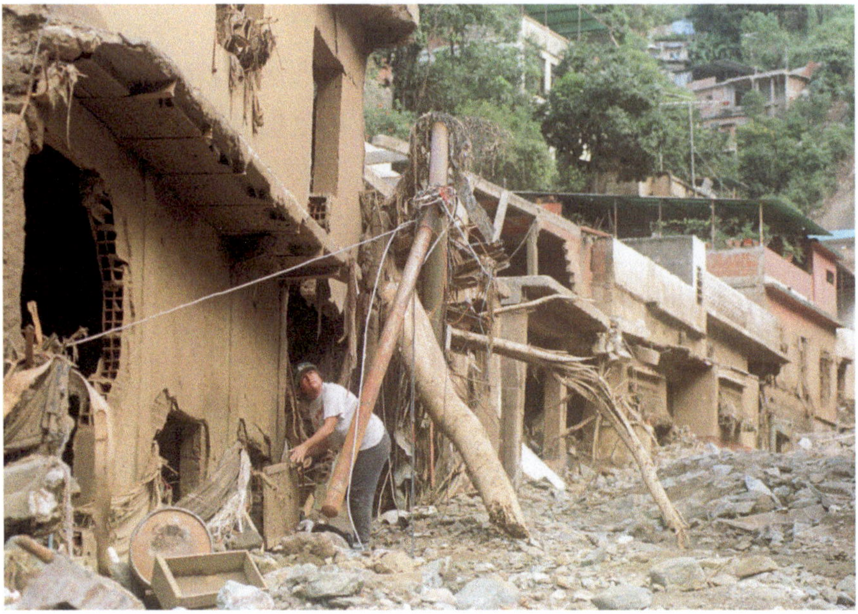

Image 5.1 Houses and streets were swept away by raging floods and mudslides. Source: Associated Press

The relief effort in the wake of the mudslides did not just include Venezuela. When the Federal Ministry of Foreign Affairs made its emergency declaration, officials appealed to international agencies and governments for aid [12]. Both national and international efforts to help those stranded and otherwise in need of help were extensive.

Throughout the devastated region, the Ministry of Foreign Affairs set up centers where victims could seek help [12]. In addition, Venezuela mobilized civil and military resources, such as Navy ships and helicopters [9]. By December 20, 4 days after the mudslides ended, Venezuelan Navy ships had transported 800 tons of drinking water to affected coastal regions [8]. When the numerous land-based shelters proved inadequate to house all who had been displaced, Navy ships were used as temporary housing [8]. Twelve thousand troops aboard Navy vessels and 25 helicopters worked in tandem to deliver supplies and rescue marooned people from the flooded areas [8]. Navy troops were not the only military personnel called into action. In several operations, President Chavez commanded 1,500 paratroopers lowered from helicopters to deliver supplies to people still waiting for rescue [13]. Such air and sea efforts were critical since roads "littered with debris and flooded by up to two feet of water" were impassable, resulting in many coastal and highland villages being completely inaccessible by land [1].

As a result of these efforts, relief workers were able to access some of the most remote villages within just 4 days of the mudslides. The victims were both relieved

18. IRIN. Tajikistan: typhoid outbreak under control. http://www.irinnews.org/report.aspx?reportid=20795. Accessed 27 June 2007.
19. Brown P. News roundup: Asia: typhoid outbreak in Tajikistan. The Guardian. Oct 24, 2003:Foreign 18.
20. ITAR-TASS News Agency. Typhoid outbreak reported in Southern Kyrgyzstan. ITAR-TASS News Agency. Oct 31, 2003:Alert.

Chapter 14
Stage Three: Internalizing

Stage three marks the beginning of emotional and intellectual deliberation about the hazard. Here, the compact group and the broader population (1) experience emotional response, (2) seek redress, (3) change normal activities, and (4) assess vulnerabilities and capacities. The onset of stage three will vary, but it is to some extent marked by the passing of immediate danger from the hazard. Emotional responses are a key feature at this point as well, but may operate differently from previous stages. On the individual level, emotions may range from acute relief, acute disbelief, sadness, and shock, to chronic mental disorders. Now the compact group, and the larger community of which it is a part, are left to consider how life must shift in a changed post-disaster world. The population also engages in a re-evaluation of vulnerability to the hazard. These reflections later motivate behaviors in the fourth stage.

Emotional responses post-disaster vary. This is well summed up in the findings of a study documenting the consequences of a fire that broke out in a dormitory of a school on the island of Vaitupu in Tuvalu. The fire resulted in the death of 18 girls locked within the dormitory and their matron who fought to rescue them [1]. In this context, the emotional response to the disaster highlighted the role of religion in the internalization of the event. Many in Vaitupu were devout Christians. Consequently the belief in God's will became a way to overcome the pain and grief surrounding the disaster [1]. In finding a purpose for the disaster, many of those mourning the death of loved ones found peace in their loss and the tragedy.

Communities unfamiliar with tragedy may also struggle to accept a disaster and their own vulnerability. Following a plane crash in 2005 in Cape York, Australia, Reverend Father George Markotsis reported that the community "grieved the 'sense of security' the tragedy had ripped from the tight knit community" [2]. In addition, Reverend Markotsis proclaimed to his congregation that the loss of the victims of the crash is accompanied by the new "reality of a disaster happening on our doorstep" [2]. Accompanying this reaction for many were a range of reactions from anger, helplessness, and pain that the disaster "happen[ed] to these special people" [2].

S. Rudenstine and S. Galea, *The Causes and Behavioral Consequences of Disasters: Models Informed by the Global Experience* 1950–2005,
DOI 10.1007/978-1-4614-0317-3_14,

The *cause* of the hazard, as well as the outcome of the hazard, may be a key determinant of the emotional response. Malicious intent (which may drive, for example, terrorist attacks) or visible institutional failure (for example, the occurrence of a chemical leak controllable by the company) may provoke a different set of emotional responses from the population. While grief for what is lost crosses lines of intent or lack thereof, in instances of malicious intent or visible institutional failure, anger and fear may be the more pronounced emotional reactions and result in individuals placing blame.

Reflection about the hazard that has passed results in the adoption of a "new normal," a new set of norms of behavior that is informed by the experience of the hazard and its immediate consequences. Affected populations may change normal activities as a consequence of the experience and an acceptance of vulnerability. Fear that they may again become a victim of such a hazard motivates some to minimize future risk by taking a variety of precautionary actions [3, 4]. After living through Norway's worst train disaster on January 4, 2000 Catriona Prebble reported to Karen Rice of *The Scotsman* that "she flees a public place if someone bumps into her by accident" due to intense feelings of vulnerability [5]. In addition, Ms. Prebble developed a fear of trains, which she faced not only out of a need to travel to Glasgow, but also out of a desire to ensure that she did not develop a "hang-up" about taking trains. Ms. Prebble described her first train ride following the crash as not "very nice" since "you are conscious of where you are sitting and how easily you can get out." [5]. As seen through Ms. Prebble's reaction to the train crash, accepting one's vulnerability in the aftermath of a life-threatening event results in subtle or obvious shifts in behavior and comfort level in various contexts. Similarly, in May 2002, residents of Calgary, even those who were not directly affected by a large fire, reported overwhelmingly being "remind[ed] of how fragile we all are" following the largest and costliest residential fire in the city's history [6].

Identification of culpabilities and vulnerabilities is central to stage three. The experience of the hazard brings community vulnerabilities and capacities to the forefront of public consciousness. Local and national parties engage in discussions about where and why the hazard and the ensuing damage occurred and did not occur. At a structural level, the post-disaster emergent norm is pieced together through urgent conversation assessing institutional vulnerabilities and capacities.

A common feature of the assessment of vulnerability is the search for a cause, or a culprit, someone, or something who is to blame for "what went wrong." In 2001, an explosion at the Brookwood mine, in Alabama, US, triggered heated debate around the cozy relationship between inspectors from the US Mine Safety and Health Administration and officials at the Jim Walter Corporation – the owner of the Brookwood mine. Mike Boyd, a union member who worked in Mine No. 5 and whose brother died in the explosion, became "vocal in criticizing the company" citing "fraternization," which resulted in "inspectors being more lenient on violations" [7]. Miners, administrators, and the community charged mining inspectors with lax safety assessments and poor enforcement of citations, arising from their socializing with mine officials, ultimately putting miners at risk [8]. Members of the United Mine Workers of America launched an investigation of the federal agency's relationship with the Jim Walter Corporation in light of the explosion [8].

References

1. Taylor AJW. Tragedy and trauma in Tuvalu. Australasian Journal of Disaster and Traumatic Studies. 2000:2. http://www.massey.ac.nz/~trauma/issues/2000-2/taylor.htm. Accessed 20 July 2006.
2. Plane crash bodies recovered as victims mourned. The Sydney Morning Herald. May 11, 2005:National.
3. Drabek TE, McEntire DA. Emergent phenomena and the sociology of disaster: lessons, trends and opportunities from the research literature. Disast Prev Manag. 2003;12:97–112.
4. Fischer HW. Response to disaster: fact versus fiction and its perpetuation: the sociology of disaster. Lanham, MD.: University Press of America; 1994
5. Rice K. Trauma goes on for city survivor of Oslo rail crash. The Scotsman. 2000:20.
6. Williamson K. Anatomy of a fire: total devastation overwhelming to firefighters, onlookers. Calgary Herald. 2002:City & Region,B1.
7. Reeves J. Questions raised about government oversight at the site of deadly mine blast. The Associated Press State and Local Wire. 2001: State and Regional.
8. Pratt T, Ellis KL. Mine violation records lacking some priority citations apparently left uncleared. Birmingham News. 2001.

Chapter 15
Stage Three: Internalizing Jefferson County, Colorado US Columbine High School Shooting – April 20, 1999

A sunny spring day ended in bloodshed at Columbine High School on April 20, 1999. Thirteen students were killed and 21 were wounded before the two gunmen, also students at the school, killed themselves. Eric Harris and Dylan Klebold waged their attack over the course of an hour, between 11:10 a.m. and 12:08 p.m., during the first of three scheduled lunch periods at the high school in Jefferson County, Colorado [1, 2].

Harris and Klebold met at 6 a.m. that morning, orchestrating and preparing their attack for 5 hours before arriving at school separately around 11:10 a.m., according to notes written by Klebold in Harris' daily planner [2, 3]. Student Brooks Brown met Harris in the parking lot used by high school juniors. As Brooks stood smoking a cigarette, Harris parked his 1986 gray Honda Civic [2] and walked toward Brooks. "I like you, Brooks," Harris said to his classmate, "get out of here" [4]. Brooks left; he was the only student warned to leave the premises before the gunfire began. Klebold, meanwhile, parked his 1982 black BMW in the southwest senior student parking lot and met Harris inside the school [2].

Once they were together, Harris and Klebold began to carry out their meticulously planned attack on the school. At around 11:14 a.m., they dropped off two duffle bags filled with explosives in the cafeteria [2, 5]. The duffle bags, placed on the floor beside two tables, blended in with the student backpacks that were always strewn around the cafeteria floor during the lunch period. By careful calculation, Harris had determined that the cafeteria would be almost full of students at 11:17 a.m. The explosives were set to go off at that peak time, but never did [2, 6].

At 11:19 a.m., a diversion Harris and Klebold had staged outside caught the attention of police and firefighters: a bomb went off between Ken Caryl and Chatfield Avenues on the east side of Wadsworth Boulevard [2]. The bomb did not fully explode. Nonetheless, as Harris and Klebold had hoped, it distracted emergency workers from what was about to happen inside the school. Harris and Klebold, wearing black trench coats, had left the school building by then and stood on its west steps. From there, they had a full view of the southwest senior parking lot, parts of the junior parking lot, cafeteria exits and entrances, and the west athletic fields [7, 8].

S. Rudenstine and S. Galea, *The Causes and Behavioral Consequences of Disasters: Models Informed by the Global Experience* 1950–2005,
DOI 10.1007/978-1-4614-0317-3_15, © Springer Science+Business Media, LLC 2012

Harris and Klebold fired their guns at students who had hoped to enjoy one of the year's first sunny spring days while eating lunch outside. Rachel Scott died. Richard Castaldo was shot several times and critically injured, but survived [2, 7].

Five students nearby heard the shots and tried to run away. Klebold and Harris turned their guns on them. Michael Johnson and Mark Taylor were hit. Taylor, debilitated, remained on the ground, while Johnson managed to flee with the others to the outdoor athletic storage shed [7].

Meanwhile, three more boys who were making their way from the cafeteria to the outdoor "smoker's pit" [2, 7] saw Harris and Klebold – and their guns. The three, Daniel Rohrbough, Lance Kirkland, and Sean Graves, assumed some sort of prank was unfolding and continued up the hill toward the gunmen. Harris and Klebold fired at them, hitting all three. Rohrbough and Kirkland lay where they fell. Klebold walked toward them and shot both again, at close range. Rohrbough died instantly. Kirkland survived [2, 7].

The injured Graves made his way back toward the cafeteria and had collapsed in the doorway by the time Klebold got there. Klebold stepped over Graves and briefly entered the cafeteria, where approximately 488 people were eating lunch. He then went back outside to rejoin Harris, who was shooting at Anne Marie Hochhalter [2, 7].

Like many of the students outside, those individuals inside the student and faculty cafeterias who first noticed Harris and Klebold initially assumed they were playing a senior prank or filming a movie for their video class. When William "Dave" Sanders, a teacher and athletic coach, entered the student cafeteria, he encountered a group of confused high-schoolers trying to figure out what was happening [2, 7]. Sanders and several school custodians quickly realized that this was more than a prank and took charge, instructing the students to move away from the windows, get down and hide under the cafeteria tables [2, 7]. Dave Sanders was shot; he died while helping students escape Harris' and Klebold's attack.

When Patricia Nielson, then a hall monitor, heard the noise, she too assumed Harris and Klebold were filming a movie. Just as she was about to yell "knock it off" [2, 7], one of them fired toward her. Bullets shattered the glass at the west entrance, where she was standing, and throughout the hallway [2, 7]. Both Nielson and a student, Brian Anderson, were injured by the flying glass and metal fragments.

When Deputy Neil Gardner of the Jefferson County Sheriff's Department was dispatched in response to a student's 911 call that a girl was injured, he expected a car accident. Instead, he was greeted with about ten gunshots in his direction from Harris, who along with Klebold had been distracted away from the school's west entrance by the lights and sirens of Gardner's squad car. Gardner quickly drew his own weapon and returned four shots toward Harris [2, 7].

Other deputies and emergency response teams soon arrived at the school where they helped Gardner secure the perimeter and monitor the students fleeing the building. Many students gathered behind patrol cars, taking cover from possible gunfire [9]. Students were evacuated one patrol car load at a time from the school premises. They were taken to secure locations for medical and mental health services.

Parents were instructed to go to these sites to find their children or to obtain information about their children's whereabouts.

By 11:29 a.m., just 10 min after the first gunshot, three people were dead and nine were injured. Harris and Klebold entered the library, one of the few places in the building still full of people. Fifty-two students from all grades and four faculty and staff members were in the library when the gunmen came in and started shooting [10]. Within 7½ minutes, Harris and Klebold killed 10 more people and injured another 12 in the library, bringing their 17 minutes total to 13 dead and 21 injured.

SWAT teams slowly secured the school, identifying possibly active bombs and evacuating nearly 2,000 students and more than 100 faculty and staff members along the way [9]. Several hundred were evacuated from the school before the SWAT teams first entered the library at 3:22 p.m. Inside, they found 12 dead, including Harris and Klebold, who "appear[ed] to have self-inflicted gunshot wounds to the head" [2].

Columbine High School was finally declared safe and secure at 4:45 p.m., putting an end to one of the three worst school shootings to date within the United States [2].

Applying Our Model of Population Behavior

As outlined in Chap. 9, population behavior after a disaster tends to follow a predictable pattern. Stages one (group preservation) and two (population preservation and altruism) (outlined in detail in Chaps. 10 and 12, respectively) explain the population's behavior immediately after the hazard strikes. Both stages focus on preservation – preserving first the compact group, those directly exposed to the hazard, and second the general population. Only after the population feels safe from the threatening hazard and ensuing disaster can individuals and groups reflect on their experiences and begin to understand what had occurred.

Stage One: Group Preservation

The behavior of the Columbine High School students, faculty, and staff throughout the attack by Harris and Klebold follows the model of population behavior suggested here. After Harris and Klebold began their attack at 11:19 a.m., students directly exposed to the gunfire confirmed the actual danger (information-seeking behavior) and then ran away from the gunmen, who were the hazard (evacuation, rational behavior). Second, students and staff still inside the school building, who could hear the developing commotion outside the cafeteria, sought information about what was occurring. They did so by peering out the windows and by speaking to students who had run back into the building (information-seeking behavior). During this period, several school custodians and one faculty member, Dave Sanders, directed the students in the cafeteria away from the windows, which looked out on the threat, and told them to hide under the cafeteria tables [2, 7]. As soon as the threat was confirmed as real, the custodians and the faculty member directed the students to leave the cafeteria through the hallways leading to the east exits of the school. It only took "seconds after the shooting began, [before] hundreds of students and teachers poured out of the school while others sought refuge inside, hiding under desks and locking themselves in bathrooms" [11]. Dave Sanders, who died from gunshot wounds suffered while helping students escape, could have evacuated the building safely instead of staying behind to help guide the students out of the cafeteria. However, his choice to stay and aid the students exemplifies group preservation behavior. Ensuring the safety of those nearby – students, faculty, and staff – was the priority.

Group preservation behavior continued until the hazard was over – the point when Eric Harris and Dylan Klebold committed suicide. Throughout the entire hour that Harris and Klebold paraded through the school, students and faculty members made several phone calls to 911 and to parents. Each call transmitted information about the attack, which helped to inform the response. Moreover, information about the gunmen was relayed by word of mouth throughout the building, at times ahead of the gunmen's movements. The spread of information allowed the students and faculty to hide and secure classrooms or, in some cases, to evacuate the school.

It is hard to know how Klebold and Harris would have reacted if they had come into direct contact with more students or teachers in the building after leaving the library massacre. As it happened, since neither killer made much effort to force his way into locked classrooms to kill more people, no one else was killed or injured. The actions of the compact group to evacuate, help one another to safety, and distribute information about the gunmen's location and actions likely played a role in limiting Klebold and Harris' contact with any more people and were likely influential in reducing the number of people who were injured or killed.

Stage Two: Population Preservation and Altruism

Contemporaneous to the actions of the compact group, a response effort was organized and implemented outside Columbine High School. The response began immediately after the first shooting when a student called 911 about a woman injured in the south parking lot. Deputy Gardner attempted to combat the hazard (the gunmen) by shooting several rounds at them. Several different service providers, including police and fire departments and emergency medical services from several districts, bomb squads, and mental health counselors had formed response teams. By the end of the day, more than 1,000 police officers and emergency medical responders were on site. These teams quickly secured the school's perimeter and remained an active part of the community for the following months, providing a wide range of services. The response teams had three common objectives: (1) terminate or gain control over the hazard (Harris and Klebold); (2) rescue and support those directly affected by Harris' and Klebold's actions; and (3) help the community at large come to terms with the event. The members of the response teams took several actions toward these goals, all of which contributed toward population preservation.

As people began evacuating the high school building, nearby police officers herded the students behind their patrol cars. The cars served as momentary shelter from sporadic gunfire within the building before the students were shuttled off the high school premises.

The Columbine Public Library and Leawood Elementary School were converted into information and service hubs – central places where evacuated students waited to be reunited with their parents and parents waited "trembling and tearful" for their children to arrive. "Hour upon hour, scores of frightened parents crowded inside and outside the library" [12]. The library remained the "command center" for months following the disaster [12].

Although Harris and Klebold were found dead, the SWAT teams remained suspicious of further danger, especially the possibility of active bombs remaining inside the school or on the school grounds. As a result, law enforcement spent seven full days searching 1,952 student lockers, all 250,000 ft^2 of the school's building, and 700 backpacks. Only after this careful inspection were the school and its surrounding areas secured and declared safe [13]. During the search, the bomb squad found 30 exploded and 46 unexploded bombs either in or around Columbine High School [13].

Stage Three: Internalizing

Internalizing refers to the population's internalization of the disaster. There are four major substages of the internalizing substage: (1) In reacting to the disaster, the *emotional response* of the population (of the individual and group) varies greatly, ranging from acute disbelief, sadness, and shock to the possible development of psychopathology or renormalization. (2) Both individuals and groups *seek redress* in which they informally allocate blame for the disaster, intending to bring justice. (3) The population begins to *address vulnerabilities*, which it identifies as underlying factors of the environment (e.g., natural, political, social, and economic) that were responsible for the disaster. (4) In direct response to the disaster, individuals or the population as a whole may *change their normal activities and routines* to fit into the post-disaster context.

The following discussion illustrates each of these sub-stages using examples from the Columbine High School community, the Jefferson County population, and the national response to the Columbine High School shooting.

Emotional Response

There was a wide range of emotional reactions to the Columbine disaster. Utter disbelief was among the more prominent and frequently voiced reactions to the

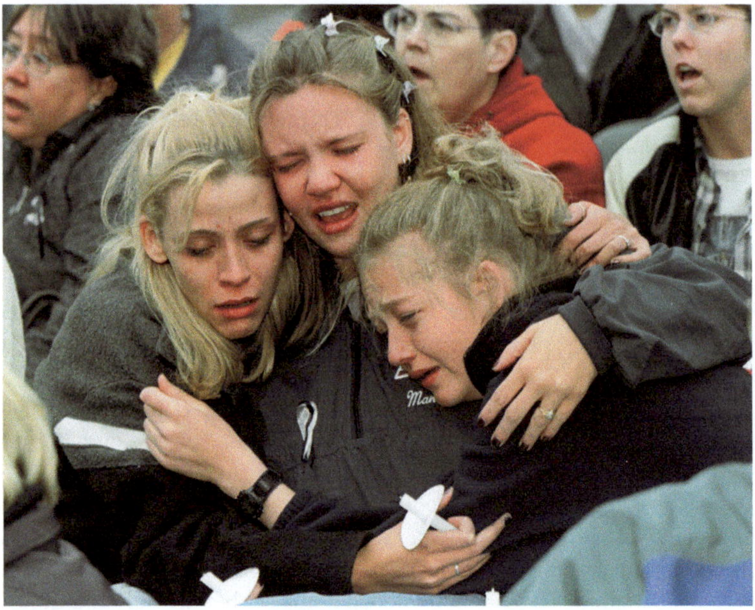

Image 15.1 High school students hug and sing at vigil in Denver. Source: Reuters

event among witnesses and victims. Klebold's and Harris' classmates, friends, and family members were not the only ones shocked by the gunmen's ability to lead double lives. Some members of the community also were paralyzed by the reality that "anyone could do this that we know" [14]. To others, it was a bad dream from which they would soon "wake up" and have things return to normal [15].

And yet for many, the Columbine tragedy was anything but a bad dream. For those who lost a family member or friend, witnessed the death of a classmate, suffered injury, or were charged with the responsibility of evacuating the scared, injured, and dead from the classrooms and halls of the high school, the horror of the Columbine shooting was unmistakably real (Image 15.1).

Many siblings and parents of those students who fell victim to gunfire reported tremendous guilt in the aftermath of the shooting. Corey DePooter's younger sister, Jena, went home for lunch on April 20. When she returned, she assumed the commotion outside the school was caused by a fire drill. She soon learned of the gunfire in the school, and thought of her brother. Corey died in the library; he was studying to "get his grades up" [16]. Jena "[wished] it had been me [Jena]…Now I'm sitting here and I don't have him anymore. I just loved him so much. I'd rather he lived than me" [16]. Similarly, Corey's mother was tormented by her son's death and believed "he wouldn't have been in the library" if she had not encouraged him to improve his grades [16].

Students who survived and saw their classmates collapse to the ground after being shot later reported rage and guilt that they did not do more to protect their classmates. Several students reported struggling to overcome feelings of responsibility for prioritizing their own safety over helping others. Bae, a sophomore at Columbine, recalled running away from the gunmen alongside another girl. The gunmen shot toward them, shattering the windows. Bae kept running, but the other girl was hit and fell to the ground. In retrospect, Bae questioned her "selfish" unconscious decision to keep running, asking, "why didn't I stop to help that girl?" [17].

Columbine survivors have reported immense relief clashing with guilt. Survivors and their families have struggled with their good fortune and their neighbors' loss. "You feel relieved when someone was found…Then you feel guilty knowing there is a parent standing at Leawood (Elementary School) and her kid is never going to come home again," offered Amy Erickson, the mother of four and neighbor of Columbine High School [18]. Parents arrived by the dozen at Leawood Elementary School in desperate search for their children. Some found their children quickly; others waited for hours. Some were told their child had been taken to a nearby hospital for medical attention. Others waited and waited in vain for their child, who would never arrive.

The events of April 20 did not just hit home for the Columbine High School community. It was personally challenging and life threatening for many of the EMS, fire, and rescue personnel who responded to the incident. Hundreds of emergency response workers were on the high school's grounds as the events unfolded. A number of teams convened outside the school to help students who had evacuated. The teams shuttled some students to safe and secure places. They also provided medical attention to the injured. The SWAT teams organized and took turns entering the building in the hope of putting an end to Harris and Klebold's violent rampage. "SWAT teams kept coming out of the school for debriefings"…"Some of them were in tears…It was very emotional to see, these guys in their combat gear. They were very affected" [19]. Jefferson County Coroner Nancy Bodelson reacted this way: "My God…what happened here?" She gazed over chairs that stood out of place and saw scarred carpet, singed by a bomb, computer screens in pieces from shotgun blasts. Then she looked down at the bodies on the floor. She could think of only one thing – her own teen-age children. "I just felt so sad," she says. "It was like I wanted to hug every one of them for their mom and dad" [19].

As with other disasters, there were reports of a variety of psychopathologies, including post-traumatic stress disorder, anxiety, and depression in the aftermath of the shootings. Jessica, a 16-year-old sophomore, was unable to sleep in her basement bedroom after the attack. Meg, a junior, had been having a "recurring" dream for weeks of "Dylan and Eric laughing," which she "[couldn't] get rid of" [20]. Others developed more severe psychopathology, which required treatment. One student, who hired Harris to work for him at a restaurant called Tortilla Wraps, "was recently admitted into a hospital for psychological reasons" triggered by the Columbine High School shooting, reported his mother, and sister to an investigator on August 10, 1999 [21]. The threat of victims developing psychopathology after the Columbine High School tragedy was well understood. More than 100 mental health counselors and psychologists from neighboring counties continued their work for a year after the disaster, debriefing rescue workers and meeting with anyone who sought help [22].

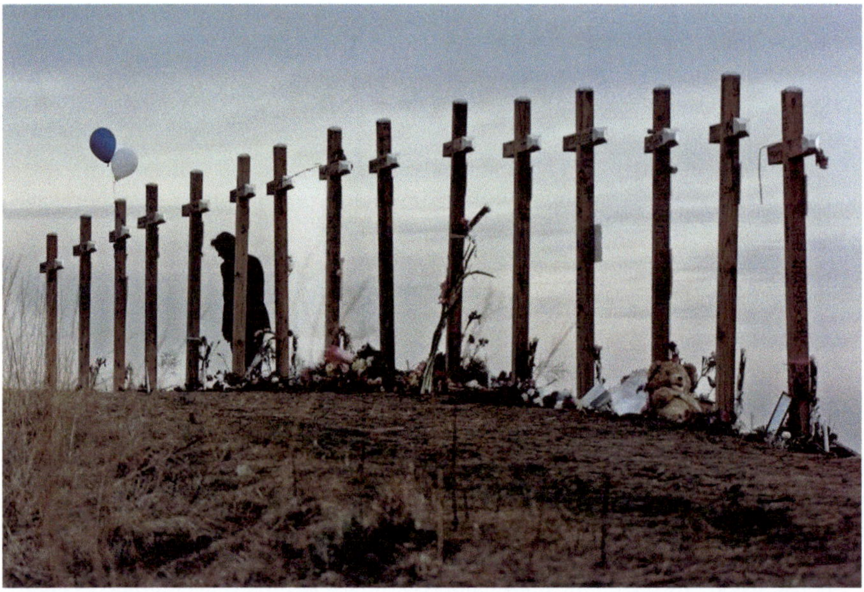

Image 15.2 15 crosses on the hill above Columbine High School in Littleton, Colorado posted in memory of those who died during the Columbine High School shooting. Source: Associated Press

Thousands of people affected by the Columbine shooting made and visited informal and formal memorials as a way "to connect in visceral ways," which provided comfort and support [23]. Within 2 days after Harris and Klebold attacked Columbine High School, Clement Park, which is across from the school, was transformed into a "mourners' mecca" [18]. It was "the site of literally thousands of informal memorials, as people from around the world came to leave signs of remembrance and support for the students of Columbine" [24]. Both residents of Jefferson County and people traveling from afar came "by the tens of thousands…clutching flowers and teddy bears, seeking God's guidance under a weeping sky…They came to share their suffering, and to lean on one another. To begin healing, celebrate courage, and pledge that Tuesday's deaths at Columbine High School were not in vain" [25]. In addition to the thousands of memorials strewn throughout Clement Park in honor and memory of the dead, 15 crosses were erected on a hilltop near Columbine High School: 13 for the victims and 2 for the killers [26]. The inclusion of the two crosses for Harris and Klebold, though controversial, was symbolic of how the "community is willing to embrace these individuals," and forgive their horrific act, Littleton resident Sharon Dunn told Tillie Fong of the Rocky Mountain News [26] (Image 15.2).

The Columbine community prided itself on its ability to pull together in the aftermath of the shooting. Despite the physical evidence of the gunmen's rampage visible in and around the high school, the community's behavior clearly demonstrated that in the words of Colorado Governor Bill Owens it "will not be beaten down" [25].

Just days after the shooting, more than 70,000 people came to mourn at the Bowles Crossing Shopping Center, which had been converted into a gathering place. In between different speeches a group of students began to yell, "We are" and another group responded "Columbine!" [25]. The spontaneous cheer was just one of several ways members of the Columbine community reclaimed their school.

As the Columbine community was living through the tragedy, leaders in Colorado and across the nation spoke words of support. Governor Bill Owens reached out to the people of Columbine, telling them: "We will stand with you shoulder to shoulder as you face your future" [25]. President Bill Clinton also offered camaraderie. "I think it is important on this day…that we continue to offer the people of Colorado, the people of Littleton, the families involved, the sure knowledge that all of America cares for them and is praying for them," he said [27].

Seeking Redress

Within hours after Columbine High School was secured, members of the community, local and national news reporters, and local and national leaders began searching for a cause of the tragedy. Shortly after the shooting rampage came to an end, news about the disaster and Harris' and Klebold's backgrounds began to appear in the media. For example, on January 30, 1998 the two teenagers were arrested for breaking into a vehicle. They were convicted and placed in a 1-year juvenile diversion program that required community service, counseling, and anger management classes [28]. After 10 months, Harris and Klebold were released early with "glowing" report cards claiming they were both "bright young men" [29, 30]. Only later did it become clear that the "juvenile authorities were deceived" [31]. For both Harris and Klebold, this was their only arrest. However, examples of Harris' disturbing behavior, including threatening the life of a classmate, Brooks Brown, and the explicit threats and angry tirades of his website were shared with his parents and reported to the Sheriff's and the District Attorney's offices before the Columbine massacre. Despite these complaints and the circumstantial evidence – which in hindsight might have been sufficient for a warrant to search Harris' house – no action was taken.

Harris' and Klebold's parents and teachers, Columbine High School's administrators, and the offices of the sheriff and district attorney all were accused by some of failing to recognize the threat the killers posed to their community. Some suggested that Harris' and Klebold's parents were inattentive, failing to recognize their sons' threatening behavior before the attack. Others suggested that their teachers acted irresponsibly when they did not report disturbing school projects, such as the gunmen's school video that portrayed them killing people or their violent and angry writing [30]. Others, however, did not blame the teachers or parents. Instead, they recognized that the gunmen skillfully masked to those around them the intensity of their anger and their willingness to seek revenge [31].

Once the public learned that a number of complaints about Harris's behavior and his website were made to the offices of the sheriff and district attorney, some people blamed the local authorities for their failure to act. Brooks Brown's father, Randy Brown, had filed a report with the sheriff's office on March 18, 1998. It contained printouts from Harris' website that indicated his will to kill [29]. The sheriff's department did not investigate the complaint or others similar to it. After the Columbine shooting, the sheriff's office stated that the complaints made a year earlier "definitely should have raised a red flag" [29]. In his defense Sheriff John Stone stated that "suspicious incidents" cannot receive the same attention as murder and rape cases; "those always take priority" [29].

While discussions in Littleton focused on the failures of the local community, significant national attention held the firearm and entertainment industries responsible for the Columbine tragedy. In a dialog between President Bill Clinton and 27 high school seniors, much blame was focused on the availability of guns to teens nationally. Of note 18-year-old Tyler Cotrone commented on teen possession of guns in Colorado and the need "to make some regulations" [32]. Similarly Tom Mauser, whose son was killed in the shooting stated "Something is wrong in this country when a child can grab a gun so easily and shoot a bullet into the middle of a child's face, as my child experienced" [33]. Others, such as President Clinton and Vice President Gore, focused on the "ultraviolent images" portrayed in television programs and video games, which "are planted like seeds in the minds of children" [34].

The Columbine High School community's values, namely its special treatment of athletes, were recognized by many as making Harris, Klebold, and many others feel like outcasts. The "school wide indulgence of certain jocks – their criminal convictions, physical abuse, sexual and racial bullying" perpetuated the "killers' feelings of powerlessness and galvanized their fantasies of revenge" [35], many parents and students believed. Yet although task forces were set up to assess the school's "jock elitism," which many argued spurred the gunmen's actions, others believed Harris' and Klebold's attack "[targeted] everyone" [36].

Addressing Vulnerabilities

The events of April 19, 1999 called attention to vulnerabilities within the Columbine High School environment and the broader national environment. Local and national discussions focused on these vulnerabilities by bringing awareness and, at times, change.

Two important vulnerabilities were recognized by the sheriff's office and the district attorney's office. First, the overwhelming number of threats and complaints reported to the sheriff's office meant that it was impossible for each threat to be investigated thoroughly [29]. Second, the sheriff's and district attorney's offices conceded their failure to appreciate the seriousness of the recurring complaints about Harris, who already had been convicted of a felony. "I suppose, in hindsight, all of us would do many things differently," Jefferson County District Attorney Dave Thomas said after the shootings [30]. In the aftermath of the shootings, many people, including the gunmen's classmates, criticized law enforcement agencies for their lack of foresight and failure to communicate effectively.

The accessibility of guns became another major concern. On May 1, 1999 people from all over the country gathered at the Colorado capitol building to protest at the National Rifle Association's (NRA) annual convention, held only 2 weeks after the Columbine tragedy. Approximately 7,000 people came together to rally against gun violence with a common underlying agenda: the desire to gain control over the availability and danger of guns. Different suggestions about how to do so included supporting child-proof locks on all weapons, banning automatic weapons, and banning all guns. The NRA refused to cancel the convention despite advance warning of the planned protest, which was part of a nationally coordinated effort to express solidarity with the victims and speak out against gun violence in 25 places throughout the country [37].

On a national level, the incident at Columbine High School fueled an ongoing discussion of the risks associated with large schools. In 1999, Columbine had approximately 2,000 students. As a result, as in most other large schools, "many students remain virtually anonymous for their entire stay" [38]. It has been suggested that the impersonal environment resulting from schools with large student bodies may amplify destructive student behavior, in contrast to smaller schools, where students are generally known by at least one adult [38–41]. This debate continues to this day.

Changes in Normal Activities and Routines

There were several noticeable changes in behavior and activities following the shooting at Columbine High School. These include: (1) interpersonal relationships within the Columbine High School community, (2) increased safety measures to prevent future incidents, both locally and nationally, and (3) postponement or cancelation of scheduled events.

The attack on the Columbine student body forced the students and faculty to confront the social structure within the school. Many argued that the school's culture had a special appreciation for jocks, which encouraged a "rift among the jocks and other factions," such as the Trench Coat Mafia, of which many believe Harris and Klebold were part [36]. Others disagreed with that perception and believed the Columbine High School community did not privilege one social group over another. Nonetheless, many felt that whatever social barriers existed prior to the shooting subsequently "disappeared." Adam Foss, a senior at Columbine High School, offered a powerful description of this change in the dynamic of the student body: "All the barriers are gone…people come up to you and throw their arms around you and tell you how they love you – students you never thought you could talk to before" [36].

Education officials responded to the attack by turning their attention to security inside school buildings. Parents and children were apprehensive about returning to school in the days after Harris and Klebold gunned down their teachers and classmates. "[A school] doesn't need to look like an armed camp…It needs to look like a place where adults are supporting their children," Superintendent Jan Hammond said in response [42]. Consequently many schools in Jefferson County did not install metal detectors. Instead inspectors assessed and heightened school security throughout the surrounding Denver area and parents volunteered to patrol school grounds and hallways [42].

News of the tragic event at Columbine High School immediately and temporarily affected scheduled events and priorities for individual actions throughout the nation. Volunteers flooded to designated areas for victims and rescue workers offered everything from mental health services to food and cellular phones. Sports teams, such as the Denver Nuggets and Colorado Rockies, canceled sporting events [43]. Even national news was put on hold when President Clinton convened a previously scheduled news conference but addressed only the events unfolding at Columbine rather than his planned agenda [27, 43].

Conclusion

The massacre at Columbine High School horrified communities throughout the United States. From the onset of Harris' and Klebold's attack on their fellow classmates and teachers, those affected sought safety and security for themselves and those closest to them. The community simultaneously worked to rescue the students and staff who were on the high school's grounds, establish necessary services to address all physical and emotional injuries from the event, and unite concerned families with their children who evacuated the building. The death of Harris and Klebold marked the end of the hazard and the beginning of the individual's attempt to internalize the tragedy that just passed. This process was not fast or predictable. Over time the community moved past the events of April 20, 1999 as students returned to high school, and yet some aspects of the community remained changed, namely a heightened sense of vulnerability that is not surprising in the aftermath of an unpredictable, unexplainable, and horrific event. The process of internalization following this event at Columbine High School – some aspects of which are still ongoing – provides powerful evidence of how a community begins to work through the emotional effects of a disaster only after the immediate threat has subsided and prior to being able to objectively seek retribution.

References

1. Stone JP, Dunaway JA. Foreword. In: Jefferson County Sheriff's Columbine High School Report. Jefferson County, CO: Jefferson County Sheriff's Office; 2000.
2. Stone JP, Dunaway JA. The Columbine High School shootings. In: Jefferson County Sheriff's Columbine High School Report. Jefferson County, CO: Jefferson County Sheriff's Office; 2000.
3. Klebold D. Jefferson County Sheriff's Office: Columbine Documents. Jefferson County, CO: Jefferson County Sheriff's Office; 1999:397. http://denver.rockymountainnews.com/pdf/900columbinedocs.pdf. Accessed 27 Apr 2007.

4. Bartels L, Crowder C. Fatal friendship: how two suburban boys traded baseball and bowling for murder and madness. Rocky Mountain News. August 22, 1999. http://denver.rockymountainnews.com/shooting/0822fata1.shtml. Accessed 19 Mar 2007.
5. Stone JP, Dunaway JA. The bombs are placed in the cafeteria. In: Stone JP, Dunaway JA, editors. Jefferson County Sheriff's Office Columbine High School Shooting Report. Jefferson County, CO: Jefferson County Sheriff's Office; 2000.
6. Stone JP, Dunaway JA. Hallway events – part 2. In: Stone JP, Dunaway JA, editors. Jefferson County Sheriff's Office Columbine High School Shooting Report. Jefferson County, CO: Jefferson County Sheriff's Office; 2000.
7. Stone JP, Dunaway JA. Findings of outside events. In: Jefferson County Sheriff's Columbine High School Shooting Report. Jefferson Country, CO: Jefferson County Sheriff's Office; 2000.
8. Jefferson County Sheriff's Office: Columbine High School Shooting Investigation Reports. Jefferson County, CO: Jefferson Country Sheriff's Office; 1999;JC-001-000112.
9. Stone JP, Dunaway JA. Deputies on scene. In: Jefferson County Sheriff's Columbine High School Report. Jefferson County, CO: Jefferson County Sheriff's Office; 2000.
10. Stone JP, Dunaway JA. Findings of library events. In: Stone JP, Dunaway JA, editors. Jefferson County Sheriff's Office Columbine High School Shooting Report. Jefferson County, CO: Jefferson County Sheriff's Office; 2000.
11. Anton M. School war zone. Rocky Mountain News. April 20, 1999. http://denver.rockymountainnews.com/shooting/0420ass00.shtml. Accessed 26 Mar 2007.
12. Abbott K. Parents wait, cry and hope. Rocky Mountain News. April 21, 1999. http://denver.rockymountainnews.com/shooting/0421par08.shtml. Accessed 21 March 2007.
13. Stone JP, Dunaway JA. Bomb summary. In: Stone JP, Dunaway JA, editors. Jefferson County Sheriff's Office Columbine High School Shooting Report. Jefferson County, CO: Jefferson County Sheriff's Office; 2000.
14. Kilzer L, Bartels L. Trench coat mafia shocked by violence. Rocky Mountain News. April 23, 1999. http://denver.rockymountainnews.com/shooting/0423thir1.shtml. Accessed 2 Apr 2007.
15. Weber B. Fear, hope fill graduation day for Columbine. Rocky Mountain News. May 16, 1999. http://denver.rockymountainnews.com/0516grad3.shtml. Accessed 3 Apr 2007.
16. Sprengelmeyer ME. I wish it had been me. Rocky Mountain News. May 2, 1999. http://www.denver.rockymountainnews.com/shooting/0502fam70.shtml. Accessed 3 Apr 2007.
17. Anton M. Death goes to school with cold, evil laughter. Rocky Mountain News. April 21, 1999. http://denver.rockymountainnews.com/shooting/0421top00.shtml. Accessed 22 Mar 2007.
18. Crowder C, Frazier D. Seeking solace. Rocky Mountain News. April 22, 1999. http://denver.rockymountainnews.com/shooting/0422mood6.shtml. Accessed 2 Apr 2007.
19. Luzadder D, Vaughan K. Inside the Columbine investigation. Rocky Mountain News. December 12, 1999.
20. Terror in Littleton: The community; Columbine students talk of the disaster and life. The New York Times, A 27. April 30, 1999.
21. Wygant SK. Interview With Kit Harmon. Southern Jefferson County; Investigation Interview Write-Up, No. 99–7625. 1999.
22. Stone JP, Dunaway JA. The victim services response. In: Stone JP, Dunaway JA, editors. Jefferson Country Sheriff's Office Columbine High School Shooting Report. Jefferson Country, CO: Jefferson Country Sheriff's Office; 2000.
23. Niebuhr G, Wilgoren J. Terror in Littleton: shrines; from the shock of violent deaths, new and more public rites of mourning. The New York Times, A 24. April 28, 1999.
24. Stone JP, Dunaway JA. The community response. In: Jefferson County Sheriff's Columbine High School Report. Jefferson County, CO: Jefferson County Sheriff's Office; 2000.
25. Anton M. Tens of thousands 'honor these children'. Rocky Mountain News. April 26, 1999. http://denver.rockymountainnews.com/shooting/0426scho0.shtml. Accessed 2 Apr 2007.
26. Fong T. Crosses for Harris, Klebold join 13 others. Rocky Mountain News. April 28, 1999. http://denver.rockymountainnews.com/shooting/0428cros1.shtml. Accessed 2 Apr 2007.

27. Romano M. Clinton calls for unity, prayer. Rocky Mountain News. April 22, 1999. http://denver.rockymountainnews.com/shooting/0422cli3.shtml. Accessed 2 Apr 2007.
28. Stone JP, Dunaway JA. Jefferson County Sheriff's Columbine High School Report. Jefferson County, CO: Jefferson County Sheriff's Office; 2000.
29. Able C, Imse A, Vaughan K. Deputy knew of Harris' threats. Rocky Mountain News. April 30, 1999. http://devner.rockymountainnews.com/shooting/0430scho0.shtml. Accessed 24 Apr 2007.
30. Anton M, Ryckman L. In hindsight, signs to killings obvious. Rocky Mountain News. May 2, 1999. http://denver.rockymountainnews.com/shooting/0502why10.shtml. Accessed 24 Apr 2007.
31. Imse A, Bartels L, Foster D. Killers' double life fooled many. Rocky Mountain News. April 25 1999. http://denver.rockymountainnews.com/shooting/0425shoo1.shtml. Accessed 2 Apr 2007.
32. Romano M. Clinton offers word of optimism. Rocky Mountain News. April 23, 1999. http://denver.rockymountainnews.com/shooting/0423pres8.shtml. Accessed 2 Apr 2007.
33. Crowder C, Frazier D. 8,000 Rally against gun violence. Rocky Mountain News. May 2, 1999. http://denver.rockymountainnews.com/shooting/0502pro40.shtml. Accessed 3 Apr 2007.
34. News Wire Reports. Clinton slams violent images. Rocky Mountain News. May 11, 1999. http://denver.rockymountainnews.com/shooting/0511task1.shmtl. Accessed 2 Apr 2007.
35. Adams L, Russakoff D. Dissecting Columbine's cult of the athlete. Washington Post, A 1. June 12, 1999.
36. Holtz R. Shootings fuel debate over 'jock elitism' at Columbine. Rocky Mountain News. April 27, 1999. http://denver.rockymountainnews.com/shooting/0427jock3.shtml. Accessed 2 Apr 2007.
37. Seelye KQ, Brooke J. Terror in Littleton: The gun lobby; protest greets N.R.A. meeting in Denver. The New York Times. May 2, 1999:1,28.
38. Raywid MA, Oshiyama L. Musing In the wake of Columbine: what can schools do? Phi Delta Kappan. 2000;81:444.
39. Cushman K. Why small schools are essential. Horace. 1997;13.
40. Cotton K. Affective and social benefits of small-scale schooling. Eric Digest, Clearinghouse on Rural Education and Small Schools [serial online]. 1996. http://ericdigests.org/1997-2/small.htm. Accessed 25 Apr 2007.
41. Raywid MA. Current literature on small schools. Eric Digest, Clearinghouse on Rural Education and Small Schools [serial online] 2003. http://www.ericdigests.org/1999-3/small.htm. Accessed 25 Apr 2007.
42. Weber B. Return to school spurs anxiety. Rocky Mountain News. April 26, 1999. http://denver.rockymountainnews.com/shooting/0426famy1.shtml. Accessed 12 Apr 2007.
43. News Staff. Grief flows across metro Denver. Rocky Mountain News. April 21, 1999. http://denver.rockymountainnews.com/shooting/0421rea14.shtml. Accessed 2 Apr 2007.

Chapter 16
Stage Four: Externalizing

Capacities and vulnerabilities determined during internalizing (stage three) become the basis for targeted action, or externalizing, in this stage. The externalizing process has two substages (1) seeking redress and (2) addressing vulnerabilities and building capacities. Post-disaster actions in this stage may vary by perceptions regarding who and what was responsible for the disaster. These in turn depend in large part on the nature of the hazard and its consequences. For example, attempts at seeking redress may be more diffuse after a natural hazard compared with a technological disaster or an act of mass violence where a central "perpetrator" is readily identified. Formal investigations and trials may be used by populations to identify and formalize redress, as well as penalize the agents of the disaster on a domestic and international scale. In disasters brought on by infectious disease outbreak, quarantine against the agent of the hazard (the visibly sick) may well be the central defense mechanism adopted by the population [1].

Seeking redress and assignation of blame emerge from the vulnerabilities identified during internalizing in general, and more specifically, from the culpability of individuals or structures that are identified during stage three. Identified "perpetrators" can be individuals, groups, or even structural features, as in the case of natural disasters. Retributive actions may be geared toward either the proximal or fundamental cause of the disaster, or both. When structural features become the primary agent considered culpable for a disaster, blame is often attributed to those charged with minimizing vulnerability, such as the engineers of a burst dam. In other cases blame may be assigned to those charged with preventing or alleviating damage, such as those responsible for controlling disease during an infectious disease outbreak.

Population consensus need not emerge for action to be taken and in many instances population consensus about a single perpetrator is never quite achieved. Different explanations for the hazard may result in an array of actions against diverse perpetrators. Actions will also vary over time – an immediate response will be different from a delayed response. Punishment for those culpable may be a legal proceeding, a war, or simply a complaint aimed at improving future action. Similarly, the magnitude of the blame and severity of punishment may lessen with temporal distance from the

S. Rudenstine and S. Galea, *The Causes and Behavioral Consequences of Disasters: Models Informed by the Global Experience* 1950–2005, DOI 10.1007/978-1-4614-0317-3_16, © Springer Science+Business Media, LLC 2012 hazard. In cases of hazards that strike large areas, it is often the case that culpability is assessed differently in different areas, with the causes of the disaster being interpreted differently by far-flung population segments.

An interesting example of differing attributions leading to different stage four actions was the 2004 floods in Nigeria. Senator Musiliu Obanikoro from Lagos Central held officials from the Land and Urban Planning Ministry accountable for permitting the construction of the Lagos Business School on a drainage channel; this was one of many construction projects approved around the vital sources of drainage throughout the flooded areas [2]. Commissioner for Environment, Mr. Tunji Bello argued that the unsanitary habits and the "[nonchalant] attitude of Lagosians to their environment" were responsible for the flooding, which resulted from "blocked drains and indiscriminate dumping of refuse into canals and drainage channels" [3]. Lagos' state Governor Bola Ahmed Tinubu called attention to a number of variables that he believed significantly enabled the flooding, one of which was the packaging of pure water in sachets, which consistently blocked drains on the streets [3].

Unlike Nigeria's 2004 floods, in which there were multiple sources blamed for the event, the Eritrean government charged the Sudanese and Ethiopian governments with sole responsibility for the terrorist attack on May 26, 2006 in Barentu. In addition, Eritrea's leaders accused Sudan and Ethiopia of creating the "axis of belligerence" alongside Yemen [4]. These accusations were made despite the lack of evidence and other suggestions by outside observers that the bombing was designed and implemented by Eritrea's own citizens [5].

Addressing vulnerabilities themselves is another substage of this period. This process assumes that there were modifiable characteristics that made the population vulnerable to the effects of the hazard and that these characteristics were known prior to the hazard but were neglected, which produced the disaster conditions. There are two nonexclusive components to this behavior: (1) enhancing group capacities from within and (2) externally led coalition building. When communities act internally to defend themselves from future disasters, disaster prevention behaviors become prevalent. Enforcement of safety regulations becomes a key issue, and sometimes tension develops when the government is unable to control population behavior and faces pressure to perform in accord with recommended post-disaster action. For example, following the 1990 Indian Airlines Airbus 320 crash, the Indian government grounded all 14 of the country's A320 aircraft pending further investigation. In addition, public critiques intensified, citing the crash as evidence for the wide-spread belief that the new Airbus 320 system was unsafe and that Indian Airlines was unprepared for flying and maintaining the aircraft [6, 7]. Jean-Claude Bidot, secretary general of the French Airline Pilots Union, called the 320 Airbus a "super complicated aircraft" that is overreliant on computers which may consequently "erode the pilots' basic flying skills," reducing the "pilots' reflexes in time of emergency" [6]. Despite widespread concern and anger regarding the risks associated with flying the Airbus 320, an Airbus spokesman state, "the Indian authorities took the decision to ground the fleet of A320s, but they appear to have done that without any justification" [6]. In addition to prevention, disaster preparedness efforts to mitigate the effects of future disasters are also typical stage four behavior. Stockpiling of resources, building physical barriers, and improvement of warning systems and communication networks may all be undertaken by affected communities to strengthen defenses in anticipation of future hazards [8].

Disaster prevention and mitigation efforts may be limited by available resources and political will. For this reason, identifying vulnerabilities is distinct from addressing them. In the flood in Nigeria, mentioned above, governing officials worked hard to reduce the flooding and address the growing needs of the population. Only after the threat of the flood subsided did attention shift to reflect on the impact of the flooding on the community. Senator Musiliu Obani-Koro stated at a news conference in Lagos, "What happened last week calls for sober reflection. All commercial and social activities were paralyzed for a whole day, while residents had difficulty moving from one place to another… Every Nigerian must be concerned about this problem [chronic flooding] and all hands must be on deck to tackle it once and for all" [9]. Moreover, aside from addressing immediate concerns, Governor Chimaroke Nnamani of Enugu State emphasized the need to implement preventative measures [10]. Of note, Governor Tinubu announced and implemented a plan that all "construction in the pathway of canals would be demolished" [11]. In addition, Commissioner Bello and Commissioner Hakeem Gbajabiamila, of Physical Planning and Urban Development, revealed plans for the McGregor canal to be dredged as a long-term solution of flooding [12].

References

1. World Health Organization. Outbreak communication: best practices for communicating with the public during an outbreak. World Health Organization; 2005; Report of the WHO expert consultation on outbreak communications held in Singapore, Sep 21–23, 2004. http://www.who.int.proxy.lib.umich.edu/csr/resources/publications/WHO_CDS_2005_32web.pdf. Accessed 31 Aug 2009.
2. Nigeria; Lagos business school may be demolished. Africa News. June 21, 2004:P.M. News.
3. Flood sacks lagos. Africa News. June 18, 2004.
4. Eritrea accuses Ethiopia, Sudan of sponsoring 'terrorism'. Agence France-Presse – English (International News). May 27, 2004.
5. BCC monitoring international reports. Ethiopian government dismisses Eritrea's claims on Barentu bomb. Global News Wire [Acc. No. A2004052768-834C-GNW]. May 27, 2004.
6. Greenhouse S. India crash receives French dispute over safety of airbus jet. The New York Times, A 8. Feb 24, 1990.
7. Hazarika S. India grounds airbus plans after crash. The New York Times, D 1. Feb 19, 1990.
8. Stallings RA, Quarantelli EL. Emergent citizen groups and emergency management. Publ Admin Rev. 1985;45:93–100.
9. Nigeria; Obanikoro seeks federal government's support to deflood Lagos. Africa News. June 22, 2004.
10. Nigeria; Nnamani wants environmental problems prevented. Africa News. June 18, 2004.
11. Vanguard. Tinubu vows to battle flood in Lagos. Africa News. June 19, 2004.
12. Vanguard. Lagos prostrates to flood. Africa News. June 18, 2004.

Chapter 17
Stage Four: Externalizing Oklahoma City, OK, US Bombing – April 19, 1995

On April 19, 1995, a bomb exploded beside the Oklahoma City's Alfred P. Murrah federal building, killing 168 people and injuring 674 [1, 2]. The blast seriously damaged surrounding buildings and smashed windows within a ten-block radius [3].

The bombing was the result of at least a year-long preparation led by Timothy James McVeigh in collaboration with Terry Nichols. At approximately 8:57 a.m. on April 19, a Wednesday [4], McVeigh implemented his plan, parking a 24-foot rented Ryder truck full of approximately 4,800 pounds of ammonium nitrate and fuel oil outside the north entrance of the Murrah building [2, 3, 5].

Within minutes the explosive mixture detonated, becoming the largest terrorist attack in the US up until that point [6]. By the time the bomb went off, McVeigh had abandoned the Ryder truck and fled downtown Oklahoma City in a yellow Mercury [7].

Although the exact chronology of McVeigh's preparations remains unclear, investigations have brought many details to light. McVeigh and a friend, Terry Nichols, began purchasing ammonium nitrate, one of the chemicals used to build the bomb, at least 8 months before the bombing [8, 9]. Nichols also bought other bomb-making materials, such as blue plastic barrels and detonators, which he stored at his house [10, 11]. Before settling on Oklahoma City's Murrah building, McVeigh visited several federal buildings around the nation in search of a target, several of his friends later testified [12].

Five days before the bombing, McVeigh checked into the Dreamland Motel in Junction City, Kansas. The same day, he reserved the Ryder truck for pickup on April 17 [6]. Investigations suggest that McVeigh and Nichols assembled the bomb between April 14 and 18 [6].

The bomb went off at 9:02 a.m. on April 19, just after the business day began in downtown Oklahoma City. More than 800 people, including 21 children who had been dropped off at the second-floor "America's Kids" Child Care Development Center, were inside the Murrah federal building [3, 5]. The majority of the other occupants were employees or visitors of the building's 14 federal agency offices [5].

S. Rudenstine and S. Galea, *The Causes and Behavioral Consequences of Disasters: Models Informed by the Global Experience* 1950–2005,
DOI 10.1007/978-1-4614-0317-3_17, © Springer Science+Business Media, LLC 2012

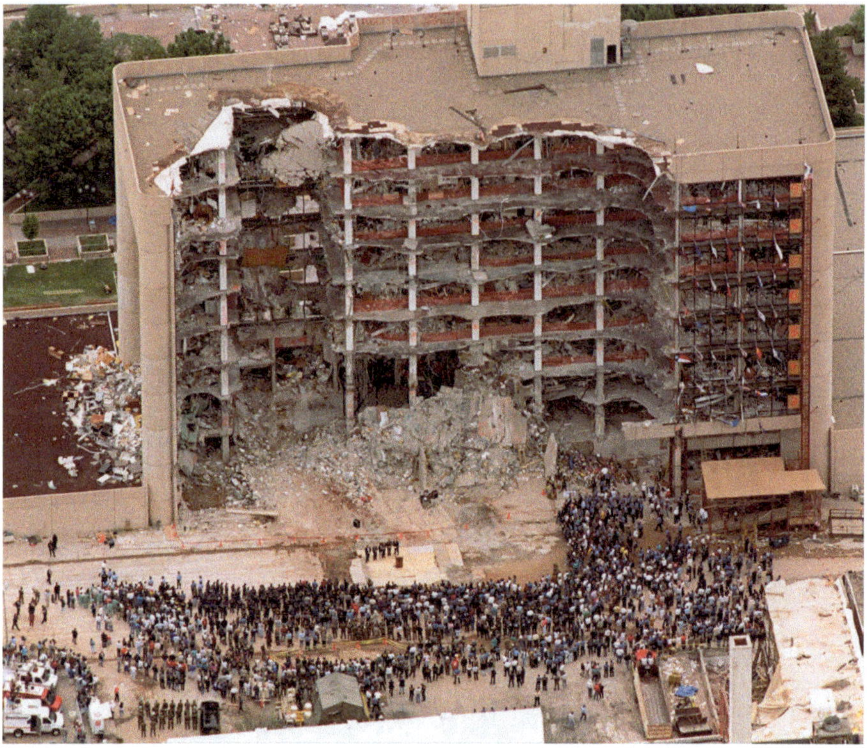

Image 17.1 The Oklahoma City Alfred P. Murrah Federal Building after the April 19, 1995 bombing. Source: Associated Press

The force of the blast caused all nine stories on the north side of the federal building "to 'pancake' into a pile of rubble" [13]. A "mushroom-shaped cloud… turned from white to black and quickly towered over the city," the result of debris from 25 damaged buildings nearby combined with the smoke emanating from burning cars [3]. The hazard came without warning and lasted only seconds. Its intensity led people throughout downtown Oklahoma City to think it was "just across the street," turning downtown into a "war zone" [14, 15]. The damaged adjacent buildings included the Water Resources Board Building, the Athenian Building, and the YMCA Building (Image 17.1).

People fled the buildings, "some in their underwear, their clothes ripped along with their skin, barefoot, walking over glass, covered in blood, dust, plaster" [16]. Some just "stumbled in shock," or, like Sharon Paulsen, who worked on the first floor of the federal building at the time of the explosion, "sat dazed on the curb" [16, 17]. Of those who escaped the collapsing buildings, some sought help nearby. Others, who were strong enough, fled, creating distance between themselves and the hazard [17].

Inside the federal building, "it felt like the world just fell in on us," some later said [17]. Others "were puzzled by the blast" [18]. Despite their confusion, people worked to free themselves and their coworkers from the rubble. Linda Logan, a secretary, who worked on the first floor, "had to dig [her] way out" while her coworkers in the Social Security office "scrambled to account for other workers" [17]. A man with his "arm blown off" entered the building and continued "attempting to help others" said witness Candy Avey, who had just parked her car outside the building [16].

As the explosion "[ripped] a huge slice from the federal building" [13], "survival depended on where the people in the building were sitting" or if, by chance, they had gotten up for coffee or to see a friend at the moment the bomb detonated [16]. "(W)e were on the west end of the building...(and) the stairwell on the southwest side of the building was open," explained Dr. Paul Heath, who was on the fifth floor at the Department of Veterans Affairs at the time of the explosion. Therefore, Heath and those around him were able to evacuate, while others perished [17].

When police in the area heard the first reports of the explosion at 9:02 a.m., they drove toward the hovering smoke and "encountered scores of walking wounded" [3]. To firefighters who arrived from the west of downtown, the Murrah building appeared intact. Initially, all they saw was severe damage to the Water Resources Board Building. As a result, initial reports suggested that the explosion occurred there. Only as the smoke cloud covering the area cleared did the firefighters first see the "gaping, debris-strewn ruin" that used to be the north side of the federal Murrah building [3]. Firefighters who entered the collapsed federal building "listened for calls for help and searched for signs of life" [3].

The Emergency Medical Services Authority first learned of the explosion at 9:03 a.m. and dispatched seven emergency medical service units to the scene. The medical teams immediately established two triage centers and began treating hundreds of victims fleeing the disaster site [5]. The rescue workers took victims rescued from the buildings to the triage areas, where they received treatment and, if necessary, were transported to surrounding hospitals. By 10:30 a.m., most of the wounded had been transported to nearby hospitals, which treated 442 people. Private physicians treated another 232 people [3].

The entire rescue effort was extensive. Soon after the explosion, the city set up an Incident Command System (ICS) to manage all incoming resources and the various rescue operations (such as federal, state, and volunteer personnel) [3]. Governor Frank Keating declared a state of emergency at 9:45 a.m. In response, personnel from federal agencies, such as the Federal Emergency Management Agency (FEMA), the National Guard, and the Federal Bureau of Investigation (FBI) began arriving downtown [5].

Rescue teams worked for 11 days in 12 hours shifts, looking for survivors [19]. Their efforts were largely in vain. One hundred and sixty-eight people were killed by the bombing; the last survivor was found in the wreckage around 7 p.m. on April 19, about 10 hours after the bombing [20]. On Sunday, April 30, the rescue operation was officially ended and transformed into a recovery operation [20]. By May 4, all but three bodies had been found, and the recovery effort, too, ended. On May 23, a Tuesday morning, the remainder of the Murrah building was imploded. Only then were the last three bodies uncovered [20].

Working in cooperation with the rescue teams, law enforcement officers conducted an extensive investigation of the crime scene. However, all the response teams (i.e., medical, firefighters, and law enforcement) agreed that the first priority was saving lives, the second was saving evidence [3]. Therefore, investigators were only allowed to scour an area for evidence after the rescue teams had thoroughly searched and secured it.

The investigators formed teams that combined federal, state, and local law enforcement officers. They worked systematically to uncover anything that might help them identify the perpetrator or the type of explosive used in the attack. By 10 a.m. on April 19, less than 1 hour after the bomb detonated, investigators uncovered two parts of a vehicle – an axle and a truck's rear end, including a license plate [21]. The identification number on the axle and the license plate led the FBI to the Ryder rental agency in Junction City and to the name Robert Kling, which was later identified as McVeigh's alias [22].

Meanwhile, as investigators closed in on an identification of the bomber, McVeigh was driving away from Oklahoma City on Interstate 35. State Trooper Charles Hanger pulled over McVeigh's car because it lacked a license plate. During the traffic stop, Hanger noticed that McVeigh was carrying a gun in a holster around his chest [22, 23]. Hanger arrested McVeigh for carrying a concealed weapon and brought him to the Noble Country Jail in Perry, Oklahoma, where he remained for 2 days awaiting a hearing [9, 22]. At the time, the local authorities did not connect McVeigh to the bombing of the Murrah building. By April 21, however, the FBI had solved the crime. Federal agents went to the Nobel County Jail and arrested McVeigh for the bombing [24, 25].

On June 2, 1997, after a 35-day trial [25] and 4 days of deliberations [26], a jury convicted McVeigh of all 11 criminal counts charged. Two days later, he was sentenced to death by lethal injection. McVeigh was executed on June 11, 2001 in Terre Haute, Indiana [26]. Nichols was convicted on December 24, 1997 and sentenced to life in prison without parole. A third defendant, Michael Fortier, also a friend and accomplice of McVeigh's, pleaded guilty to a minor firearms charge and testified against Nichols and McVeigh. In exchange, he received a more lenient sentence of 12 years in prison and a $200,000 fine [25].

Applying Our Model of Population Behavior

As outlined in Chap. 9, population behavior after a disaster tends to follow a predictable pattern. Stages one (group preservation) and two (population preservation and altruism) (outlined in detail in Chaps. 10 and 12, respectively) explain a population's behavior immediately after a hazard strikes. The first stage focuses on preserving the compact group, those directly exposed to the hazard. The second focuses on the preservation of the general population. Only after the population feels safe from the threatening hazard and ensuing disaster can individuals and groups reflect on their experiences and begin to understand what occurred (stage three, internalization, as discussed in Chap. 14).

Stage One: Group Preservation

The actions of the people trapped inside the Murrah federal building and the surrounding buildings illustrate the group preservation stage. Few initially understood the cause of the explosion. Some assumed that the rumbling and destruction were caused by "a tornado or something" [27]. Others, including the approaching firefighters, believed the Water Resource Building had exploded [3]. Regardless, after the detonation individuals stood up, looked around, and quickly realized the enormity of the situation. "The most concerning thing about my office is… there is an office to the right of me and an office to the left of me, and (after the explosion) there was just nothing there. It was bare," said Jim Hargrove, who worked on the third floor of the Murrah federal building [18]. He and others inside quickly evacuated.

Getting out of the building was not easy. Because doors were jammed shut and stairwells were destroyed by the rubble, some people "tied curtains together to escape…lowering themselves through windows" to the ground [18]. Many people were trapped under collapsed concrete blocks and entwined in the rebars, bars of steel that had reinforced the building [16]. Victims who were unharmed or only slightly injured "seemed more concerned not with their own injuries but with the fate of their friends" [16]. As a result, "coworkers struggled to rescue one another" before finding their way out of the building [16].

Stage Two: Population Preservation and Altruism

While the victims inside the Murrah building were helping each other evacuate the collapsing building, rescuers outside were organizing and news of the explosion was spreading. "Virtually everyone in the county learned of [the bombing] instantly" [28]. "Rescuers swarmed from all corners of the city and eventually the surrounding states" [16]. Moreover, over a 100 doctors and nurses arrived at nearby hospitals and triage centers to volunteer services within hours of the explosion [16]. For more than 2 weeks, rescue workers toiled "nonstop" in 12 hours shifts in "debris and unstable conditions," pulling victims out of the rubble [28]. More than 12,000 people participated in the rescue and recovery efforts [29].

People who could not offer medical or rescue services "searched for ways to help" [16]. Hundreds "waited in line for 6 h to donate blood" [16]. Many others responded to requests made by various organizations for donations of items such as baby formula, clothing, and batteries [16]. In addition to individual donations, businesses such as McDonald's and Domino's Pizza donated food. Within 24 hours of the explosion, the Midsouthwest Foodservice Convention and Exposition donated more than 10,000 meals. As a result, rescue workers and victims had more than enough food and supplies.

Around the country, people "sat gazing at the television, immobilized by the shock" and desperate to learn more about the source of the explosion and the victims [28].

At John Marshall High School in Oklahoma City, administrators set up television sets in the school's cafeteria "so students could keep up with the bombing news during lunchtime" [30]. Radio, television, and newspapers such as The Oklahoman provided in-depth reports on the rescue operations, the city's recovery process, the suspects, and the resulting trials and sentencing hearings. The national media also catered to the desire for information; the New York Times published a series called "Terror in Oklahoma" and Time magazine, among others, published frequent reports and updates.

Stage Three: Internalizing

The Oklahoma City bombing happened in an instant. The subsequent rescue and recovery operations lasted over 2 weeks. During this period survivors of the bombing, victims' families, rescue workers, and people around the city and the nation were exposed to constant media reports and footage of the event as well as a national dialog centered on the victims and on those responsible for the bombing. The overwhelming nature of the disaster led to a wide range of reactions to and explanations for the tragedy.

Terrorism on US soil was almost nonexistent before the Oklahoma City bombing. As a result, there was widespread disbelief and shock that such a horrendous act could "happen here" in America. Terrorism, for many Americans, was associated with South America and the Middle East, not with "America's Heartland" [31–33]. Many veterans of the Vietnam War compared the bombing of the Murrah building to their combat experiences in Vietnam, calling downtown a "war zone" [15]. Thu Nguyen, a veteran of the Vietnam War, whose son was in the day care center in the Murrah building at the time of the bombing reflected on the disaster stating, "[Vietnam] was war. These are children. This is not war. This is a crime" [16].

While many people throughout the country struggled to accept the possibility of a "homegrown terrorist" [34] in the US, thousands of doctors, nurses, firefighters, law enforcement officers, and federal investigators were on the front lines helping injured victims, unearthing the bodies and body parts of adults and children and desperately searching for a lead to the perpetrators.

Rescue workers and law enforcement officers worked to uncover victims and evidence of how the crime occurred. The process was both physically and emotionally exhausting. Rescue workers were "haunted by being unable to save people" [35]. As firefighters searched, they were "afraid," aware that some of the people trapped under the collapsed building were children [21]. Rescue workers "wept as they cradled them [children], limp and weightless," unable to "bear to look down at the children in their arms," witnesses later recalled [16]. The grueling work began to affect the rescue workers within days of the bombing. They "[showed] signs of stress, both physically and emotionally" [16]. Supervisors instituted plans for workers to see mental health counselors throughout the rescue operation to help them "cope with what they were seeing" [16].

A national dialog around assignation of blame for the attack and aiming to address vulnerabilities within Oklahoma City started almost immediately after the bombing. For example, before Timothy McVeigh was identified and arrested for masterminding and carrying out the bombing, many public statements accused Arab extremists and overseas terrorists [36–38]. Once McVeigh was apprehended, national attention shifted to him, with public exclamations of anger and revenge, such as "kill the creep" and "baby killer" [39].

Meanwhile, national figures and agencies began to document the insufficient security surrounding various government buildings and the architectural weaknesses of a number of federal buildings throughout the nation. In particular, two facts surfaced regarding the Murrah federal building. First, several experts suggested that the building's "architecture might have made it more vulnerable to bomb damage than other designs" [40]. Second, 2 months before the bombing, "federal officials considered the building so safe that they decided to assign only one security officer there" [41], a decision questioned in hindsight.

Stage Four: Externalizing

Externalizing consists of actions taken by the population (1) against those responsible for the hazard and (2) to prevent the consequences of similar hazards in the future.

Actions Taken Against Perpetrators/Those Responsible

The Oklahoma City bombing was an intentional and "devastating attack on innocent people" [42]. Within hours of the bombing of the Murrah federal building, agents from the FBI arrived in downtown Oklahoma City desperate to uncover evidence that would help them identify the perpetrator. Tensions arose between rescue workers and the investigators responsible for sifting through the crime scene. While both sides appreciated that the priority was to save lives, the growing desire to seek justice led to frustration as investigators were prohibited from searching parts of the building until rescuers checked for victims [21]. Nonetheless, investigators soon uncovered parts of the Ryder truck that McVeigh used to deliver the bomb, which led them quickly to McVeigh. Politicians and national figures voiced their support for the FBI, promising: "(W)e will use all our resources available to us on the federal level to apprehend who did this" [42].

The federal investigation in its entirety took more than 2 years to complete. Evidence quickly led to McVeigh and his two known accomplices, Nichols and Fortier. Still, investigators were unable to connect the planning of the bombing to any large organizations, including any of the well-known right wing militias with which McVeigh had periodically been affiliated. Nevertheless, President Bill Clinton, among others, continued to associate the bombing with antigovernment militia groups. "How dare you call yourselves patriots and heroes?" Clinton asked of militia groups in a May 1995 speech. "…There is no right to resort to violence when you don't get your way. There is no right to kill people. Those who claim such rights are wrong and un-American" [43] (Image 17.2).

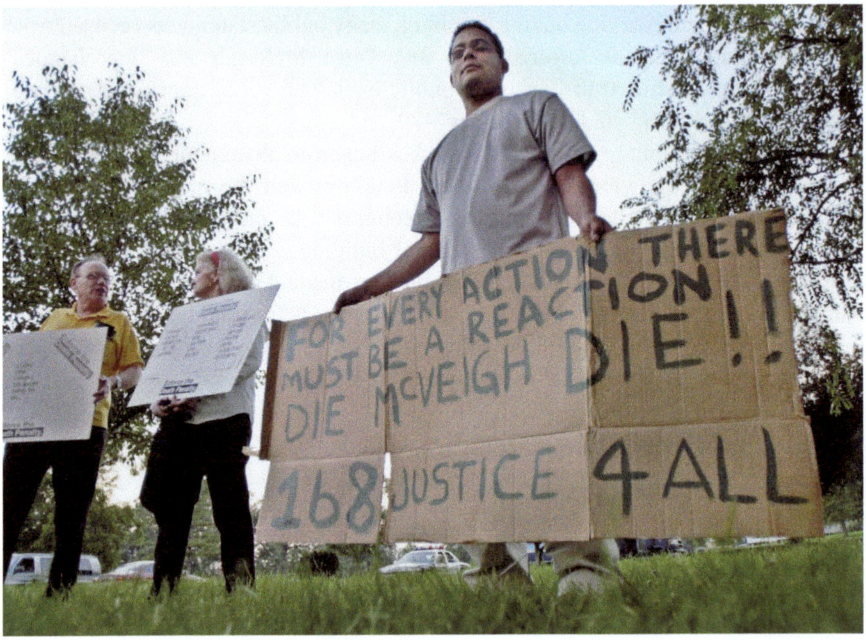

Image 17.2 Supporters of the government's execution of McVeigh as the sentence for the Oklahoma City Bombing. Source: Associated Press

McVeigh was executed on June 11, 2001, more than 6 years after his attack on the Murrah federal building. That afternoon, President George W. Bush spoke briefly to the nation, saying, "(t)his morning the USA carried out the severest sentence for the gravest of crimes. The victims of the Oklahoma City bombing have been given not vengeance, but justice" [44]. While many victims and families of those who died agreed with President Bush, others considered McVeigh's execution "revenge" for a horrible crime [45], capturing the not infrequent difference in reaction to disasters, and the subsequent pursuit of retribution.

Addressing Vulnerabilities

The attack on a US federal building exposed a number of vulnerabilities across the country that put US cities and the federal government at risk. Two of these vulnerabilities were insufficient security and the accessibility of bomb-making materials. Governing bodies and private corporations worked to raise awareness and to create new guidelines and legislation in response to concerns about these vulnerabilities.

The Oklahoma City bombing taught the country that "the USA is no longer impervious to that urban terrorism which their West Europe allies have known for a long time" [46]. Local, state, and federal officials were forced to develop new ways to ward off domestic terrorism. For example, the FBI increased its domestic terrorism teams by several hundred and officials from all levels of government acknowledged that "communication between different law enforcement agencies and jurisdictions is vital" [47, 48].

The ease with which the bomb was placed outside the Murrah federal building forced the federal government and the governing boards of each individual federal building across the country to address security surrounding and inside the buildings. "President Clinton ordered tightened security at federal buildings," insisting that officials "take any necessary precautions," White House spokesman Mike McCurry said on April 20, 1995, the day after the bombing [49]. The US Marshal Service prohibited parking in front of federal courthouses [38]. In Denver, security guards were assigned to day-care centers [50]. In June 1995, the US General Services Administration released a detailed evaluation of security and risks in more than 1,300 federal buildings [50]. In addition, Clinton stated his intention to pass new counterterrorism legislation "giving federal agents vast new authority to plant wiretaps and electronic listening devices" [41].

Along with the increased security measures nationally, a group of architects, engineers, government officials, and politicians turned their attention to the architectural design of existing and future federal buildings. "(T)he biggest structural engineering lesson learned from the Oklahoma City bombing was the need to improve the structure's ability to sustain local damage and remain standing" [32], said Todd Rittenhouse, one of the people advising the General Services Administration. No security measure can succeed in preventing all terrorist attacks; when an attack occurs, localized damage is inevitable. However, improving a building's architecture to prevent "progressive collapse" can minimize the scope of the disaster [32].

Accessibility to firearms is a common debate at public forums and congressional hearings. Public debate over the threat of ordinary substances that are also ingredients in explosives occurs less often. McVeigh used ammonium nitrate, a fertilizer used by farmers, to make the bomb that blew up the Murrah building. Therefore, despite only sporadic pressure from forensic experts to regulate the sale of ammonium nitrate, broader public awareness of "the threat posed by these legal and abundant fertilizers" occurred following the Oklahoma City bombing [51, 52]. After much debate and several other incidents of ammonium nitrate being used in explosives, the Department of Homeland Security sponsored legislation in March 2007 that presents "guidelines and allows us to monitor ammonium nitrate transactions without unduly burdening legitimate users or keeping it out of the commercial market" [51].

Conclusion

Arresting McVeigh, establishing his guilt, and carrying out his sentence of the death penalty were critical to the population's sense if retribution (and for some, revenge) for the tragic event on April 19, 1995. Other efforts to ensure that such an attack would never again succeed against government property furthered one's sense of safety. As a result, a number of security measures were taken to restrict access to federal buildings and minimize architectural risks as prevention against possible future attacks. These actions, all aspects of externalization, demonstrate how the US moved to minimize feelings of vulnerability to hazards by actively eliminating past threats and reducing the possibility of future weakness.

References

1. The City of Oklahoma City Document Management Team. Forward. In: The City of Oklahoma City Document Management Team, editor. The city of Oklahoma City: Alfred P. Murrah Federal Building bombing. April 19, 1995. Oklahoma City, OK: Fire Protection Publications; 1996.
2. Manzi C, Powers MJ, Zetterlund K. Critical information flows in the Alfred P. Murrah Building bombing: a case study. Washington, DC: Chemical and Biological Arms Control Institute; 2002; Special Report 3.
3. The City of Oklahoma City Document Management Team. Part 1: shock and response, April 19, 1995, 9:02–11:22 a.m. In: The City of Oklahoma City Document Management Team, editor. The city of Oklahoma City: Alfred P. Murrah Federal Building bombing. April 19, 1995. Oklahoma City, OK: Fire Protection Publications; 1996. p. 9–21.
4. The Oklahoman. The Oklahoma City bombing: the history. The Oklahoman. http://newsok.com/bombing/history/. Accessed 7 May 2007.
5. The Oklahoma Department of Civil Emergency Management. After action report: Alfred P. Murrah Federal Building bombing. April 19, 1995. Oklahoma City, OK: Department of Central Services Central Printing Division; Executive summary. http://www.ok.gov/OEM/Publications_&_Forms/index.html. Accessed 14 May 2007.
6. Collins J. The weight of evidence. Time Magazine. April 28, 1997. http://www.time.com/time/magazine/article/0,9171,986240,00.html. Accessed 14 May 2007.
7. Bernstein EM. Terror in Oklahoma: the overview; evidence linking suspect to blast offered in court. The New York Times, A 1. April 26, 1995.
8. Gleick E. Detours on the trail of the bombers. Time Magazine. May 22, 1995. http://www.time.com/time/magazine/article/0,9171,982961,00.html. Accessed 14 May 2007.
9. Johnston D. Terror in Oklahoma: the overview; F.B.I. issues alert for 2 more sought in bombing inquiry. The New York Times, A 1. May 2, 1995.
10. Nichols Guilty on all Charges in Oklahoma City Bombing Trial. http://www.pbs.org/newshour/updates/nichols_05-26-04.html. Accessed 25 May 2007.
11. Belluck P. Terror in Oklahoma: in Kansas; agents find possible link to bombers at lake site. The New York Times. May 2, 1995:18.
12. Gleick E. Something big is going to happen. Time Magazine. May 8, 1995. http://www.time.com/time/magazine/article/0,9171,982899,00.html. Accessed 27 May 2007.
13. Lackmeyer S, Zizzo D. City struggles with shock of deadly bombing. The Oklakhoman. April 20, 1995. http://newsok.com/bombing/article/1175507/?template=bombing/main. Accessed 14 May 2007.
14. Ottley T, McVeigh T, Nichols T. Oklahoma bombing bad day dawning. http://www.crimelibrary.com/serial_killers/notorious/mcveigh/dawning_1.html. Accessed 14 May 2007.
15. Ross B, Perry J, Gilliland P. Quotes. The Oklahoman. April 20, 1995.
16. Gibbs N. The blood of Innocents. Time Magazine. May 1, 1995. http://www.time.com/time/magazine/article/0,9171,982867,00.html. Accessed 14 May 2007.
17. Palmer G. I had to dig my way out. The Oklahoman. April 20, 1995. http://newsok.com/bombing/article/1175351/?template=bombing/main. Accessed 14 May 2007.
18. Gilliland P, Sutter E. Whatever it was, it was awfully cruel. The Oklahoman. April 20, 1995.
19. The City of Oklahoma City Document Management Team. Part IV: sustaining the effort. April 22–April 29, 1995. In: The City of Oklahoma City Document Management Team, editors. The

city of Oklahoma City: Alfred P. Murrah Federal Building bombing. April 19, 1995. Oklahoma City, OK: Fire Protection Publications; 1996. p. 51–67.
20. The City of Oklahoma City Document Management Team. Part V: recovery, healing, and remembrance. April 30, 1995–March 1, 1996. In: The City of Oklahoma City Document Management Team, editor. The city of Oklahoma City: Alfred P. Murrah Federal Building bombing. April 19, 1995. Oklahoma City, OK: Fire Protection Publications; 1996.
21. Belluck P. Terror in Oklahoma: at ground zero; Federal agencies' priorities grating as time wears on. The New York Times, A 21. April 26, 1995.
22. Ottley T. License Tag Snag. http://www.crimelibrary.com/serial_killers/notorious/mcveigh/snag_2.html. Accessed 15 May 2007.
23. The Associated Press. Officer responsible for McVeigh arrest shares his story. Oklahoman. July 23, 2005.
24. Walsh E. One arraigned, two undergo questioning. Washington Post. April 22, 1995.
25. Oklahoma bombing chronology. Washington Post. http://www.washingtonpost.com/wp-srv/national/longterm/oklahoma/stories/chron.htm. Accessed 25 May 2007.
26. Novak V, Shannon E. Playing for a stay. Time Magazine. June 11, 2001. http://www.time.com/time/magazine/article/0,9171,1000062,00.html. Accessed 25 May 2007.
27. Defrange A. I thought it was a tornado. Oklahoman. April 20, 1995.
28. Lii JH. Terror in Oklahoma: the scene; for searchers, exhaustion grows as hope fades. The New York Times. April 30, 1995:1,27.
29. Healing the Pain: Newshour with Jim Lehrer Transcript. http://www.pbs.org/newshour/bb/remember/jan-june00/ok_4-19.html. Accessed 27 May 2007.
30. Killackey J. Schools helping students cope with tragedy. Oklahoman. April 20, 1995.
31. Applebome P. Terror in Oklahoma: weapons; increasingly, extremism is heavily armed. The New York Times. April 30, 1995:27.
32. Prendergast J. Oklahoma City aftermath. Civil Eng. 1995;65:42–5.
33. Nadel BA. Oklahoma City: Security Civics Lessons. http://www.buildings.com/Articles/detail.asp?articleID=3623. Accessed 25 May 2007.
34. Smolowe J. Enemies of the state. Time Magazine. May 8, 1995.
35. Healing the Pain. http://www.pbs.org/newshour/bb/remember/jan-june00/ok_4-19.html. Accessed 25 May 2007.
36. Ottley T. Innocence Lost. http://www.crimelibrary.com/serial_killers/notorious/mcveigh/lost_3.html. Accessed 25 May 2007.
37. Lacayo R. Rushing to bash outsiders. Time Magazine. May 1, 1995. http://www.time.com/time/magazine/article/0,9171,982892,00.html. Accessed 25 May 2007.
38. Candiotti S. Wounds Remain for Bombing Victims Six Years Later. http://www.cnn.com/SPECIALS/2001/okc/stories/overview.html. Accessed 25 May 2007.
39. Gleick E. Who are they? Time Magazine. May 1, 1995. http://www.time.com/time/magazine/article/0,9171,982868,00.html. Accessed 25 May 2007.
40. Wald ML. Terror in Oklahoma: the building; design could have been another enemy. The New York Times, A 27. April 28, 1995.
41. Labaton S. Terror in Oklahoma: security; before the explosion, officials saw little risk for building in Oklahoma City. The New York Times, A 19. May 2, 1995.
42. Godfrey E, Parker J. Heartland easy target, McCurdy says. Oklahoman. April 20, 1995.
43. Adams K, Lofaro L, Quinn K, Rubin JC, Sanders AL, Urquhart S. The week. Time Magazine. May 15, 1995.
44. Landsberger C. The End of the Line for Inmate McVeigh. June 11, 2001. http://www.time.com/time/nation/article/0,8599,129972,00.html. Accessed 25 May 2007.
45. Pooley E. Death or life? Time Magazine. June 16, 1997. http://www.time.com/time/magazine/article/0,9171,986526-3,00.html. Accessed 25 May 2007.
46. Schmemann S. Terror in Oklahoma: security; overseas, Oklahoma City bombing is seen through prism of experience. The New York Times. April 30, 1995:1,28.
47. Anti-Defamation League. A Decade After Oklahoma City Bombing, Domestic Terrorism Threat Still Looms. http://www.adl.org/learn/extremism_in_the_news/Anti_Government/okc_10years_40805.htm. Accessed 25 May 2007.

48. Anti-Defamation League. Oklahoma City Bombing 10 Years Later: Lessons Learned. http://www.adl.org/ADL_Opinions/Terrorism/OKCity_oped.htm. Accessed 25 May 2007.
49. Bockiewicz RE. Federal building security tightened. Oklahoman. April 20, 1995.
50. Lacayo R. How safe is safe? Time Magazine. May 1, 1995. http://www.time.com/time/magazine/article/0,9171,982869,00.html. Accessed 25 May 2007.
51. Committee on Homeland Security. Ammonium Nitrate Legislation Introduced. http://homeland.house.gov/issues/index.asp?ID=192&SubSection=0&Issue=0&DocumentType=0&PublishDate=0. Accessed 25 May 2007.
52. Gorman C. The bomb lurking in the garden shed. Time Magazine. May 1, 1995. http://www.time.com/time/magazine/article/0,9171,982870,00.html. Accessed 25 May 2007.

Chapter 18
Stage Five: Renormalization

Renormalization is the fifth and final stage of our post-disaster population behavior model. It progresses through three substages (1) cultural adaptation to post-disaster circumstances, (2) normalization of vulnerability, and (3) domination of new modes of behavior. Through the renormalization process, behaviors which emerge during the aftermath of the disaster are absorbed into the daily fabric of life of those affected by these events.

First, hazards and subsequent disasters influence the evolution of social systems [1]. Societies must adapt to conditions produced by hazards and disasters to survive. Although cultural interpretation and reactions to disasters vary, incorporation of disasters into daily life, as well as political, economic, and social organization, is a cross-cultural phenomenon [2]. This results in the establishment of cultural shifts, creating a "new normal." For example, despite attempts to use the same architectural designs and materials to rebuild communities after an earthquake, many towns near Pradielis, Italy, suffered repeated damage from earthquakes between 1968 and 1978. A senior government official noted "the second earthquake taught us that we could not rebuild with our hearts… we needed technology" [3]. Further rebuilding accounted for the risk of earthquakes by modifying traditional architectural designs with more earthquake-resistant structures. Another example is represented in how governing officials addressed and implemented new and ongoing safety measures following the 1977 train derailing in Granville, Sydney, Australia. The disaster worsened when the derailed train collided with a bridge, which collapsed after its support beams gave way [4]. Following the disaster the Granville Memorial Trust was established. The Trust sponsors annual memorials at the site of the crash, and is instrumental in identifying rail safety concerns and encouraging fines for noncompliance with safety measures [4, 5].

Second, the experience of the disaster forces recognition of vulnerability, and negotiation for survival creates a collective acceptance of this vulnerability. For example, a population culturally familiar with sporadic and unpredictable terrorist bombings, residents of Ambon, Indonesia, "were back to their daily activities as if the tragedy had never taken place" within a day of a bombing near the Maluku

S. Rudenstine and S. Galea, *The Causes and Behavioral Consequences of Disasters: Models Informed by the Global Experience* 1950–2005,
DOI 10.1007/978-1-4614-0317-3_18,

Governor's office [6]. The persistent expectation of vulnerability influences new dominant modes of behavior. The degree to which populations affected by a disaster may continue to expect vulnerability depends on the amount of information provided to the public, and is largely fueled by mass media. These expectations also arise from the behaviors exhibited during the internalizing stage, which are at this point, becoming normal.

Third, the renormalizing process concludes when new modes of behavior, motivated by the disaster experience, become dominant. Over time, daily life for individuals and organizations slowly modifies to accommodate new behaviors until these new behaviors become normal. New emergency procedures and equipment are adopted within an organization in response to the cause of a hazard. For example, after the 1975 Moorgate Tube Crash in London, the National Rail introduced the Moorgate Control, which served as protective stopping devices to ensure that trains slow down appropriately so as not to crash into the end of tube tunnels [7]. Similarly, following the Granville train derailing described above, underlying structural vulnerabilities resulted in increased attention to railway maintenance and improved standards over time [4].

References

1. Fritz CE, Marks ES. The NORC studies of human behavior in disaster. J Soc Issues. 1954;10:26–41.
2. Gigerenzer G. Out of the frying pan into the fire: behavioral reactions to terrorist attacks. Risk Anal. 2006;26:347–51.
3. Fleming LB. Italy seeking to learn from past quake mistakes. Los Angeles Times, D 8A. July 26, 1978.
4. Commuter train wrecked, Granville, Sydney, Australia. http://danger-ahead.railfan.net/accidents/granvill.htm. Accessed 20 July 2007.
5. Granville memorial organizers forced to beg. The Daily Telegraph. Jan 15 2007.
6. Indonesia's ambon back to normal after bomb blast: report. Xinhua General News Service (World News; Political). Apr 4 2002.
7. Moorgate tube crash – 28th February 1975. http://www.fireservice.co.uk/history/moorgate.php. Accessed 12 Sept 2009.

Chapter 19
Stage Five: Renormalization South Africa Traffic Accidents – December 23, 1998 and September 22, 1999

South Africa's roads have historically been among the deadliest in the world. In 1995 there were 8,335 fatal collisions (500,233 total road traffic collisions) throughout the country, resulting in 10,256 deaths [1]. Although not all of South Africa's road accidents constitute a disaster, as defined by the criteria presented in Chap. 2, many do. S'Bu Ndebele, Kwazulu-Natal Member for Executive Council (MEC) for Transport (cabinet at the provincial level), suggested that South Africa's problem was founded on "passive acceptance of unacceptable and indeed criminal actions on our roads to blatant disregard for the law" [2]. Through this case study we see how a society works to address underlying vulnerabilities in the face of a recurrent series of repeated disasters, and consequently how new behaviors emerge, exemplifying stage five as discussed in Chap. 18. Because this case study examines multiple car accidents within the context of a history of frequent traffic accidents, it will not follow the same format as our previous case studies, which portrayed individual hazards located in time and space. We will offer an anecdote about two specific car accidents that are in our dataset as a backdrop to discussing the systematic programs that South Africa put in place to address a long history of unsafe roadway behavior.

The severity and consequences of South Africa's road accidents ranged dramatically from single- car crashes (e.g., into a light post or a pedestrian) with no to few casualties, to multiple car pile-ups leaving dozens injured and dead. Traffic accidents occurred on roads throughout the country; however, N1, a national road between Cape Town and Johannesburg became famous for the most horrific accidents, thus adopting the nickname "the death strip" [3]. One such head-on collision occurred between a fully occupied bus and a large truck pulling two trailers loaded with fertilizer on December 23, 1998 [4]. Twenty-one people were killed, four of whom were children, and 19 were injured [5]. The crash "left bodies, limbs, and belongings strewn over the road" [6]. Piet Meyer, Western Cape's MEC of transport, stated after visiting the crash site that "I have never seen such a horrific accident" [5] (Image 19.1).

Another example was a crash between a luxury bus and a lorry on N1 on September 22, 1999 leaving 11 people dead and approximately 34 injured. According

S. Rudenstine and S. Galea, *The Causes and Behavioral Consequences of Disasters: Models Informed by the Global Experience* 1950–2005,
DOI 10.1007/978-1-4614-0317-3_19,

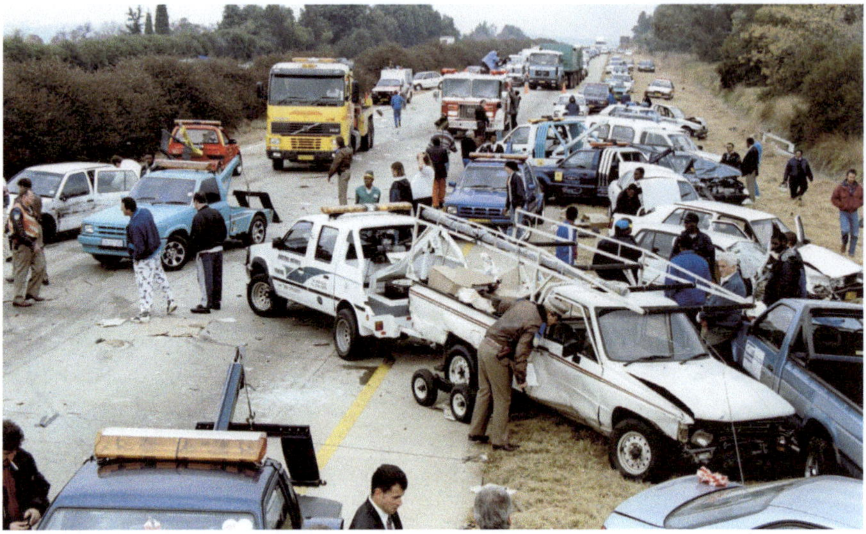

Image 19.1 A 27-car accident in 1997 on a South Africa highway in Johannesburg. Source: Reuters

to passenger statements, the lorry swerved across the road, into oncoming traffic. The bus driver tried to veer to avoid the approaching truck, but the vehicles collided, hitting on their left sides. The bus rolled onto its side; some passengers were flung outside while others were trapped within and beneath the bus [7]. Rescue workers and medical teams rushed to the accident site and worked to identify victims, remove them from the wreck, and transport those injured to medical facilities for proper care [8]. As rescue efforts got underway at the crash site, Intercape Mainliner Bus Company initiated a 24 hours phone service for people seeking information on friends and family suspected to be on the ill-fated bus [9]. News of the accident spread quickly throughout the region. Political figures expressed "shock and horror" [9]. But the familiarity of such events also triggered frustration and anger that such accidents, despite great national efforts, continued to occur on a regular basis: "We have to get to the bottom of these accidents. If there are shortcomings in road signs, or if driver fatigue played a role, or the roadworthiness of the vehicles, whatever the cause may be, such accidents have to be stopped" stated Gerald Morkel, Western Cape Premier, to news agencies after calling for an urgent investigation into the bus–lorry disaster [10]. Minister of Transport, Dullah Omar, noted that "many innocent people are losing their lives through negligence and recklessness" and appealed to drivers throughout the country to "respect and obey traffic laws and to exercise extra caution and tolerance on the road" [11].

After years of accepting the occurrence of ghastly and preventable traffic accidents on South Africa's main highways, the mid-late 1990s brought a new energy aimed at addressing the underlying causes of the accidents: excessive and consistent speeding, drinking and driving, irresponsible pedestrian behavior, driving for extended and unsafe periods of time, and driving without legal licenses. Despite speed limits on all South African roads, which were in line with speed limits on similar roads internationally, speeding had become a normal and acceptable pattern of behavior among drivers as well as law enforcement, who under-regulated the main highways [12]. Similarly, driving after drinking had become an acceptable behavior. Lawrence Barrett, a Pretoria traffic criminology expert reported, "Everyone drinks. After work, you have a couple beers...you play sport, you have a beer or three...and then you drive home" [13]. Despite efforts among traffic police to mitigate some of these behaviors, their efforts fell short of reducing the prevalence of accidents. One significant reason for this was that South Africa's traffic police were only scheduled to work from 8 a.m. to 5 p.m. Monday through Friday despite government reports documenting that 65% of all accidents occurred on weekend evenings [14].

Pedestrians contributed to the accidents. The majority of pedestrians killed by moving automobiles lived in shantytowns along the highways and often crossed the roads as they moved from their homes to neighboring communities, water holes, or small markets. Pedestrians, hard to identify on dark highways by speeding and often intoxicated drivers [15], constituted more than a third of those killed during these accidents [16].

In response to an annual increase in accidents and a notable increase between Christmas 1996 and Easter 1997, the national government, with the help of provincial and local governing bodies, implemented Arrive Alive, a program modeled after a successful road safety initiative in Victoria, Australia. Arrive Alive's mission was to address the underlying causes of South Africa's road accidents by changing the population's attitude about road safety [17–19]. Paul Mashatile, the Member for Executive Council of Transport in Gauteng, supported Arrive Alive, stating, "We would be ignoring our duty if we continued to allow people to drive or walk alongside a road while under the influence of alcohol, maintain a speed too high for circumstances, not wearing seatbelts, drive an unroadworthy vehicle or committing other serious moving offenses" [18]. Despite being a national program, resources were unevenly distributed throughout the country, predominately being used in Gauteng, KwaZulu-Natal, and Western Cape, three of South Africa's provinces, in which 75% of the nation's recorded road accidents and 53% of fatalities occurred [20]. The program's aim was to reduce the number of accidents by 5% annually.

Arrive Alive was designed to be implemented in three stages from October 1997 until October 1998, overlapping with holiday periods where road travel had historically been more dangerous (December through April). In addition to consistent attention to speeding and driving under the influence, each stage introduced a new level of prevention, education, and enforcement. Specifically, stage one, lasting from October 1997 through January 1998, targeted seatbelt compliance, stage two, February 1998 to April 1998, addressed driver fatigue, and stage three, implemented in October 1998, tackled pedestrian safety [14, 21, 22] (Image 19.2).

Immense resources were used throughout Arrive Alive's campaign. Categories of spending included: equipment, overtime pay (to encourage traffic officers to work during peak accident times, evenings, and weekends), communication (e.g., public health announcements), and training/information. In sum, 50.0 million Rand (R) was spent in stage one, R10.0 million in stage two, and R43.0 million in stage three.

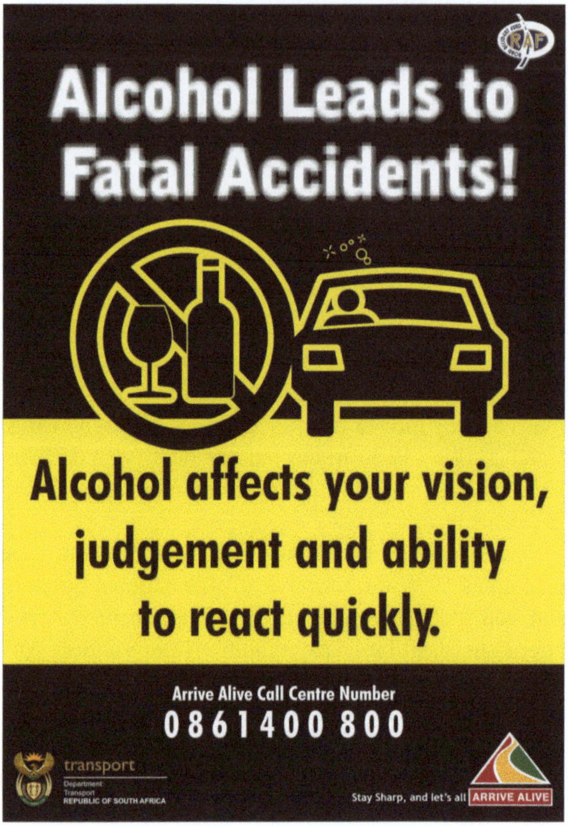

Image 19.2 An Arrive Alive poster designed to target drunken driving, a leading determinant of fatal accidents. Source: Arrive Alive

The success of Arrive Alive was founded on government and administrative support. In addition, corporate, organizational, and citizen support were essential to the integration of the program into the population's daily life. Within the three-stage implementation of Arrive Alive, dozens of corporations demonstrated public support of the program's mission by financing the program and instituting independent public awareness campaigns that highlighted the risk behaviors targeted by Arrive Alive. For example, South African Breweries invested R4.2 million in their own campaign, which adorned the Arrive Alive logo, and R1 million was donated to the Arrive Alive campaign [12]. Without these contributions it is likely that Arrive Alive would have not succeeded at changing the patterns of road behavior [12]. The integrated movement to address the chronic nature of traffic accidents was central to addressing "a culture in which road users realize their co-responsibility to preventing accidents" and where "every citizen has a role to play in putting an end to road deaths" [18].

Arrive Alive was successful in reducing the number of road accidents and fatalities. Provisional statistics in December 1998 (the beginning of Arrive Alive's stage three) documented a 14.4% reduction in accidents and 10.9% reduction in fatalities since the program's start [23]. By the end of stage three, Arrive Alive had become "a recognizable brand" [16]. Despite these improvements, the number of accidents and fatalities remained high, which is of little surprise given the state of South Africa's roads prior to Arrive Alive. Therefore, while a good and successful start, it was not sufficient to address the chronic difficulties and embedded risk behaviors facing South Africa's concerned government and citizens. Consequently, energy was invested in broadening Arrive Alive's mission, programs, and strategies to create a 7-day a week and year-round long-term road traffic safety program. The result was Road to Safety Strategy, 2001–2005. This strategy constituted nine projects, each responsible for a different aspect of road traffic management: Arrive Alive; Driver Fitness; Vehicle Safety; Pedestrian Safety; Fraud and Corruption; Traffic Information Systems; Fleet Operations Management; Professionalism in the Traffic Fraternity; and National Traffic Information and Call Centre [16].

During the years that Arrive Alive and Road to Safety were implemented and gaining momentum, road traffic in South Africa was on the rise. More vehicles were on the road, 4.07% between 2003 and 2004, and the average annual daily traffic increased 3.14% from 2002 to 2003 and 5.15% from 2003 to 2004 [24]. Fatal road accidents increased from 1998 to 2002, but began to show a steady annual decrease of a rate of 8.63 in 2004 [24]. A similar trend is visible in the number of road fatalities per 100 million vehicle kilometers, decreasing steadily between 2002 and 2004 at a rate of 10.44 [24].

Permanent change in population's behavior in response to trauma is a process that evolves at various paces and is triggered by direct and indirect exposure to hazards. Unlike a single unique hazard that affects an entire population, large road accidents affect a defined group of individuals at any one time. Arrive Alive and Road to Safety were national campaigns that branded road accidents as a national disaster rather than smaller and contained accidents. Moreover, these campaigns were both targeting established drivers at the time they were implemented and new drivers.

The ability of Arrive Alive and Road to Safety to institute a national consciousness for road safety is a tribute to an integrated effort to attack the risk behavior on South Africa's roads. Subsequent programs, such as National Road Safety Strategy, which launched in 2006, have continued these efforts in collaboration with a growing campaign within the population to improve road safety [25].

References

1. Department of Transport. Transport Statistics 2001. http://www.transport.gov.za/library/docs/stats/2001/statistics.html#2.4. Accessed 23 May 2008.
2. Ndebele S. Speech delivered by Kwazulu-Natal MEC for transport, S'Bu Ndebele, at the editors' briefing during the launch of the Asiphephe Road Safety 2000–2001 Campaign, Durban. October 31, 2000. http://www.kzntransport.gov.za/speeches/2000/31-10-2000.htm. Accessed 31 May 2007.
3. South African Press Association. 11 dead, 34 injured in bus-lorry accident in Karoo. Global News Wire. Sept 22, 1999.

4. RoundUp: 21 killed in South Africa road accident. Deutsche Presse-Agentur (International News). Dec 23, 1998.
5. Toll in South Africa bus crash rises to 21. Agence France-Presse – English (International News). Dec, 23 1998.
6. South African Press Association. Owners of ill-fated bus company pledge to help crash victims. Global News Wire. Dec 23, 1998.
7. 11 Killed, 29 injured in bus crash in S. Africa. Agence France-Presse – English (International News). Sept 22, 1999.
8. South African Press Association. At least ten people killed in bus accident near Laingsburg. Global News Wire. Sept 22, 1999.
9. South African Press Association. Karoo accident: inquiry number set up. Global News Wire. Sept 22, 1999.
10. South African Press Association. Karoo smash: premier calls for urgent investigation. Global News Wire. Sept 22, 1999.
11. Omar D. Statement from the Minister of Transport, Dullah Omar, on the bus crash on N1 between Prince Albert and Laingsburg. http://www.transport.gov.za/comm-centre/pr/1999/pr0922.html. Accessed 15 Nov 2006.
12. Maharaj M. Speech delivered by The Minister of Transport, Mac Maharaj, at the National Launch of Arrive Alive: Phase 3 – Johannesburg International Airport, 23, November 1998. http://www.info.gov.za/speeches/1998/98b24_drive19811408.htm. Accessed 28 Nov 2006.
13. S. African traffic fatalities reach a peak. Agence France-Presse – English (International News). Jan 10, 1997.
14. Department of Transportation. Arrive Alive – a closer look. Contributory factors in road crashes. http://www.transport.gov.za/projects/arrive/closer.html. Accessed 13 Nov 2006.
15. Schiller B. Highway slaughter is just a way of life. The Toronto Star (Insight, A 23). Apr 4, 1991.
16. Omar AM. The road to safety: an update on the implementation of the road to safety strategy – 20 November 2002. South Africa: Department of Transport; 2002:1–23. http://www.info.gov.za/view/DownloadFileAction?id=70264. Accessed 20 June 2007.
17. Maharaj M. Speech by the Minister of Transport, Mr. Mac Maharaj: Launch of 'Speed Kills' for the Arrive Alive Campaign, 4 November 1997 at Green Point Stadium, Cape Town. http://www.info.gov.za/speeches/1997/111758297.htm. Accessed 28 Nov 2006.
18. Department of Transport. Arrive Alive: road deaths are no accident. Stringent measures against traffic offenders. http://www.transport.gov.za/library/docs/robot/arrive.html. Accessed 17 Jan 2007.
19. Road Safety in South Africa: Historical Perspective. http://www.arrivealive.co.za/history.aspx?title=. Accessed 8 Mar 2007.
20. Department of Transport. Positive Effects of Arrive Alive Campaign Felt Nationwide, October 29. http://www.info.gov.za/speeches/1997/10310W26497.htm. Accessed 28 Nov 2006.
21. Road Safety in South Africa, Historical Perspective. http://www.arrivealive.co.za/history.asp?mc=history&nc=aasa&title=historical. Accessed 8 Mar 2007.
22. De Beer EJH. Evaluation of the Arrive Alive Phase 6 Campaign: December 2001 to July 2002. Pretoria, South Africa: CSIR Transportek; 2002;CR-2002/73:i-48.
23. Maharaj M. Statement by the Minister of Transport, Mac Maharaj, on Road Traffic Statistics for December 1998. http://www.info.gov.za/speeches/1999/99108_arrive99_10003.htm. Accessed 28 Nov 2006.
24. Road Traffic Management Corporation. Road Traffic and Fatal Crash Statistics, 2003-2004. http://www.arrivealive.co.za/document/2004-CrashBook-N.pdf. Accessed 2 Aug 2010.
25. Road Safety Strategy in South Africa. http://www.arrivealive.co.za/pages.aspx?i=1346. Accessed 2 Aug 2010.

Part IV
Our Models: Applying a Public Health Perspective

Chapter 20
Two Models, One Disaster
New York City Terrorist Attacks on the World Trade Center – September 11, 2001

September 11, 2001 was a day unlike any previously known in the United States. At 8:46 a.m. and 9:03 a.m. two hijacked commercial passenger airliners crashed into the North and South towers of the World Trade Center (WTC) in New York City. Smoke filled the sky of lower Manhattan, fire lapped at the windows of the towers, and steel, glass, and office supplies fell through the air to the ground. Within 90 minutes of the first plane crashing into the North tower, both towers collapsed. Over 2,800 people died and thousands were injured at the WTC, which encompassed nearly 16 acres in lower Manhattan. Of those who died, 343 were firefighters, 23 were New York police officers, and 37 were Port Authority police officers, all of whom were involved in the rescue efforts following the initial attack [1–4] (Image 20.1).

Two other hijacked commercials passenger planes crashed that day, one into the Pentagon and the other – intended to hit the White house or Capitol Building – into a field in southern Pennsylvania. Rescue workers and response agencies in the affected regions acted quickly and saved many lives, but the devastation was great and paralyzed the country and much of the world.

Entire books are written about the events of the September 11, 2001 terrorist attacks. In this chapter, we limit our discussion to the events that occurred in New York City. We use the event to illustrate the underlying factors that contributed to the disaster, consistent with the model we describe in Part 2 of this book, and then to illustrate population behavior after the disaster, consistent with the model we describe in Part 3. Since the literature on the topic is vast, we use here illustrative examples to illuminate each part of the discussion.

S. Rudenstine and S. Galea, *The Causes and Behavioral Consequences of Disasters: Models Informed by the Global Experience* 1950–2005,
DOI 10.1007/978-1-4614-0317-3_20, © Springer Science+Business Media, LLC 2012

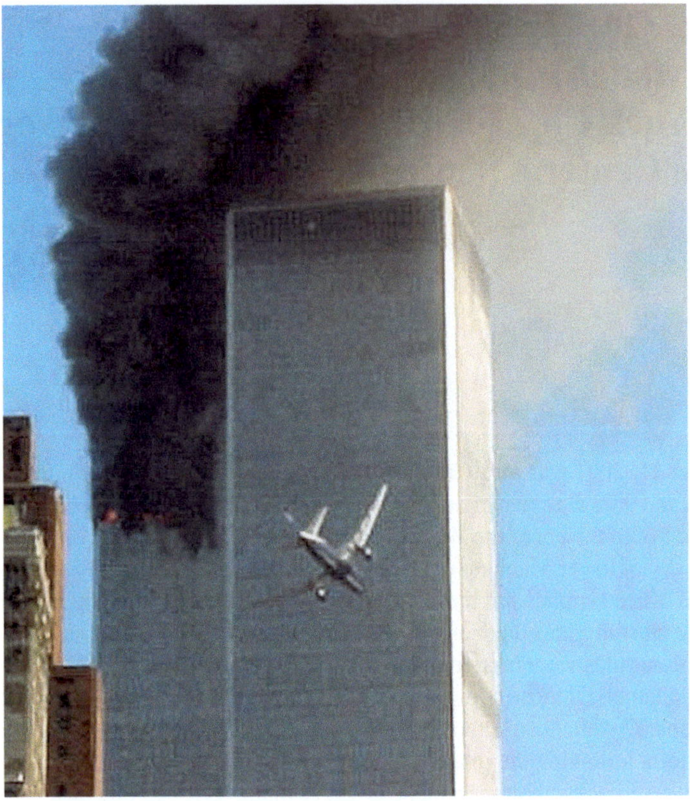

Image 20.1 Minutes after the North tower was attacked the second hijacked plane headed for the South tower on September 11, 2001. Source: Associated Press

Model One: Causes of Disasters

Capacities

New York City's first response teams were ill equipped and inadequately trained to effectively tend to a disaster of the proportions of September 11, 2001 [5]. However, the responses of the fire and police departments represented an enormous effort and unquestioned heroism by members of both the departments. Within minutes of the first plane hitting the North tower of the WTC, three of New York City's primary emergency response agencies were fully engaged in assessing the extent of the threat and addressing the needs of those directly affected by the ensuing disaster. By 8:50 a.m., just minutes after the first plane hit the North tower of the WTC, the New York Police Department Aviation Unit assigned two helicopters to investigate extraordinary options for evacuating persons trapped in the upper floors of the high-rise. On the ground, NYPD mobilized 22 lieutenants,

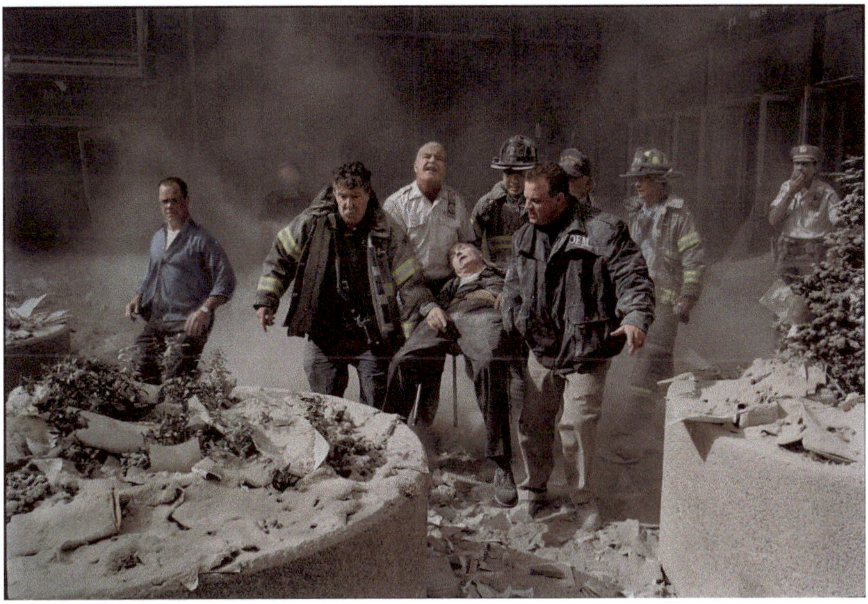

Image 20.2 Emergency response personal carry an injured man from the World Trade Center after both towers collapsed. Source: Associated Press

100 sergeants, and 800 police officers from all over the city to attend to the WTC disaster at 8:58 a.m. Two minutes later 21 engine companies, 9 ladder companies, 4 elite rescue teams, 2 elite squad companies, the department's only Hazardous Materials Response Team, and significant numbers of support staff were dispatched to the World Trade Center by the Fire Department of New York (FDNY). These teams comprised 235 firefighters; many more would become involved throughout the rescue efforts. Emergency Medical Services (EMS) was busy setting up triage centers surrounding the WTC buildings. Assisting these city agencies, the Port Authority police, many of whom were stationed in the vicinity of the WTC buildings, began rescue and evacuation efforts on the ground floors of the buildings and in the Port Authority Trans-Hudson (PATH) station that was situated below the WTC buildings [5].

There are innumerable examples of how the response agencies' efforts were integral to the survival of civilians within the towers. For example, firefighters accessed the 22nd floor of the North tower and rescued trapped civilians. Other responders from the FDNY, NYPD, and the Port Authority Police Department (PAPD) carried to safety individuals physically unable to evacuate the South and North towers. Despite the collapse of the South tower, FDNY, NYPD, and PAPD responders continued to assist civilians evacuating the towers [5] (Image 20.2).

Response teams continued steadily night and day to identify and rescue those individuals still alive, but caught in rubble, after the towers' collapse. The rescue effort was painstaking, discouraging, and challenging. As massive machines were used to disentangle the rubble from the mounds of steel, concrete, and glass that were the WTC towers, emergency response workers assessed, with waning hope, for signs of life within the debris. The capacity to launch the "largest rescue operation in the city's history" in less than 20 minutes and the sustained efforts to rescue individuals speaks to the depth of capacity in NYC's emergency services [6].

Vulnerabilities

Despite having four trained and resourceful emergency response departments and an organized oversight committee within the Office of Emergency Management (OEM), the terrorist attacks exposed substantial vulnerabilities that hindered the success of the various rescue efforts and contributed to the death of many. We focus here only on emergency evacuation procedures.

As rescue efforts unfolded, confusion over proper evacuation procedures developed among the tower's occupants. Future investigations into the mayhem surrounding the evacuation of both towers revealed startling evidence suggesting the inadequacy of the evacuation procedures provided to the WTC employees prior to September 11, 2001. In particular, no forethought was given to evacuation plans for individuals located on floors above potential fires and consequently prevented by the hazard from proceeding down stairs or elevators [5].

On September 11, 2001, hundreds of employees on the upper floors of the North and South towers were trapped, unable to pass through the rubble and fire caused by the planes' impact. Despite the evacuation plans drafted and implemented after the 1993 WTC attack, evacuation procedures for occupants on floors above a potential fire were deficient. Rooftop evacuations, a previously used strategy for evacuating stranded individuals during fires, had been prohibited in the years following the 1993 disaster. This change in evacuation procedures and the new policy that doors leading to the roof would be locked were never communicated to the WTC employees [5]. Consequently, individuals who were trapped either above the fire caused by the plane's crash or on floors where infrastructural damage blocked access to stairwells and elevators waited to no avail for communication about alternate evacuation procedures or for the arrival of help.

The 9/11 Commission Report analysis of the evacuation highlights the consequence of the inadequate evacuation procedures for those trapped [5]. Of those who died in the disaster and who were not first responders, security or fire personnel, volunteer civilians who ran into the buildings to help others, or on the two planes that hit the towers, only 5% were located below the impact zone and ensuing fire. Therefore 95% of those who died were present on floors above the impact zone, and consequently were trapped [5]. The disproportionate number of individuals who died above the impact zone marks the centrality of faulty evacuation plans as a vulnerability contributing to the September 11, 2001 disaster.

Intermittent Stressors

Evacuation on September 11, 2001 was difficult, frustrating, and impossible for many. Compounding the physical challenges to evacuation, and the long-term vulnerability represented by the inadequate evacuation plans, communication problems throughout the rescue efforts were an intermittent stressor that hindered attempts at informing the building's occupants of evacuation instructions as well as interagency communication about evacuation options for the building's inhabitants. For example, at 8:57 a.m. the FDNY ordered a full evacuation of both the towers. However, due to poor inter- and intra-agency communication throughout the next hour, 911 operators and FDNY dispatchers continued instructing civilians above and below the impact zones not to evacuate. In addition, 911 operators and FDNY dispatchers did not know that rooftop evacuations were not possible and consequently did not inform those located above the impact zone who called in for help that their only evacuation option was to descend [5].

Intermittent Protectors

After the North tower was attacked, occupants of the South tower initially did not know what had happened. Many believed the South tower was affected while others knew that the South tower was intact and that the incident was occurring in the North tower. The idea that another plane would strike the South tower was unfathomable, and as such, building personnel instructed South tower occupants to stay in their offices [5]. Despite instructions from building personnel and general confusion, many occupants chose to evacuate the building on their own accord. Particularly, in an illustration of the role of unanticipated intermittent protectors, officials in large companies such as Morgan Stanley, occupying 20 floors, on their own initiative ordered their employees to evacuate. Had these individuals not acted collectively and independent of the orders from the Deputy Fire Safety Director, even more lives would have been at risk just minutes later when the South tower fell victim to attack.

Model Two: Behavioral Consequences of Disasters

From the moment that the first plane hit the North tower, and for years after, those directly affected by the disaster and the country as a whole have followed a trajectory of behavior that illustrates the model of population behavior proposed in this book. To offer a complete review of the population's response to the September 11, 2001 terrorist attack over a number of years would require its own book. In this chapter, we limit ourselves to using examples for each stage of our model of population behavior after disasters.

Stage One: Group Preservation

Acts of group preservation were common on September 11, 2001. An estimated 17,000 people were in the WTC when the planes crashed into the towers [7]. Many people with an available evacuation route instinctively or at the urging of company managers (e.g., Morgan Stanley, as described in the above intermittent protector section) and response officials evacuated quickly. In the midst of fear and confusion, many put their own lives at risk in an effort to ensure the safety of friends, colleagues, and strangers. Harry Ramos, at the risk of his own life, chose to remain in the WTC to try to save the life of a stranger – both individuals died. John Paul DeVito organized his staff and led them out of the building to safety [8].

In addition to the decision to evacuate, firefighters who passed descending civilians on stairwell B reported being "impressed with the composure and total lack of panic shown by almost all civilians" [9]. In turn "many civilians were in awe of the firefighters and found their mere presence to be calming" [9]. Although first responders such as firefighters, were not in the towers when the planes crashed, they became members of the compact group as soon as they entered the towers and faced the same threat to their lives as those civilians within the towers. In fact, despite some orders to evacuate the towers many firefighters proceeded to ascend the tower's stairs with the determination to save those remaining in the buildings.

There were several examples of attempts to collect information as a way to inform compact group behavior in stage one. Civilians within the two towers frantically called emergency response operators (911) to inquire about what had happened and how they should proceed. Others called friends or family for information that served to guide their decision to evacuate the buildings [10].

Stage Two: Population Preservation and Altruism

New York City official agencies and residents worked to help those directly affected by the attack on the WTC. For many New Yorkers on September 11, 2001, helping consisted of walking together on the streets away from the disaster zone [11]. For emergency response providers, however, helping in the immediate aftermath of the disaster meant quickly traveling towards the WTC site and contributing to the rescue effort. Despite communication problems, and the growing infrastructural risks, individual responders entered the WTC towers to assist civilians trapped inside.

Large numbers of New Yorkers and residents of the surrounding area went to lower Manhattan hoping to help in any way possible. "People waited for hours to give blood, they delivered food to hospitals, they offered help if they had any to give" [11]. Grace Spence was quoted by Mirta Ojito of The New York Times as saying, "I'm here to do whatever…I can hold hands, listen to stories, sweep streets, whatever" [12]. By the evening of September 12, 2001 the New York Blood Center announced it had a sufficient supply of blood and would postpone collecting further donations

[12]. Skilled volunteers, such as psychologists, engineers, medical professionals, and construction workers were bused into lower Manhattan to assist the first responders. However, many of these professionals were not needed due to the large number of volunteers already at the site.

Companies, such as NY Waterway, designated all 24 of their boats to serve as "floating ambulances from piers in Lower Manhattan and others to go to Hoboken, New Jersey, Hunts Point in Queens, and the Brooklyn Army terminal" [13]. As NYC transit shut down, thousands of civilians were left to walk home or were stranded by waterways from getting home. In response, the Circle Line Tour Company and NY Waterway created a ferry service to New Jersey, Queens, and Brooklyn [13]. Private citizens who owned boats shuttled people around town. Waterways became a critical way of getting those stranded home safely and those injured to hospitals in neighboring communities that were less burdened than those in Manhattan.

Americans from across the United States and much of the world worked to support and aid those affected by the tragedy. Mirta Ojito of *The New York Times* wrote of a young couple who drove to Manhattan from Ithaca, NY to offer professional services to children, "I'm willing to assist children in any way, to counsel, to reassure them, to play games with them, to let them know they are loved and cared for" [12]. Generous acts of altruism were abundant in the days and weeks following September 11.

Information gathering was also essential at this stage. As people sought out ways they could be helpful, many were trying everything possible to learn if their loved ones, who may have been in the WTC, were safe. Throughout the world, those who knew individuals in New York sat anxiously waiting to hear of their safety. Suzanne Combrink, who lives in South Africa, told of the anguish she and her family felt for 3 hours as they waited to hear if her brother's son, who was in NY for work on September 11, was safe [14]. Not long after the first plane hit the North tower the cell phone system was overwhelmed by the abundance of calls being made on cell phones. The internet became a medium for communicating and satisfying the need for connection and information [15]. Bill Shunn, a writer and computer programmer in Queens, NY created a website to allow individuals in NY to enter their names in order to alert people that they were safe [16]. Others sat glued to the TV or radio desperate for information about those responsible or affected by the attack and the progress of the rescue efforts. Caryn James of the New York Times wrote on September 12, 2001, "The images were terrifying to watch, yet the coverage was strangely reassuring simply because it existed with such immediacy, even when detailed information was scarce…On a day of death, television was a lifeline to what was happening" [17].

Stage Three: Internalizing

There have been several studies that have documented the emotional reactions to the September 11, 2001 terrorist attacks as these attacks were internalized by the population. Pew Research Center for the People and the Press released survey findings on September 19, 2001 that since the attacks 79% of women and 62% of men reported being depressed, and 40% of women and 26% of men were experiencing difficulties sleeping [18]. Within 2 weeks of the disaster, doctors' offices reported an increase in people seeking attention for complaints of "generalized aches and pains, which could be a virus or could be malaise of the soul trying to react to this" [19].

Trends in mental health following the attack on the WTC were evaluated by government agencies, clinicians, and researchers. In a study of Manhattan residents at 5–8 weeks after the attack, Galea et al. [20] reported 8.8% of the population met criteria for post-traumatic stress disorder (PTSD) and 57.8% reported at least one symptom of PTSD in the past month. In 2007, the New York City Health Department released findings that suggest that one in eight (12.4%) rescue and recovery workers met criteria for PTSD 3–4 years after the disaster [21]. Emotional reactions to the terrorist attacks were widespread; a study administered by the National Organization for Research at the University of Chicago (NORC) found that 4–6 months after the disaster, 25.2% of the national population worried about safety. At the same time point, 42.5% of the nation felt angry, 21.1% felt depressed, and 8% reported symptoms consistent with PTSD [22]. In addition, this same study found that in response to the September 11 attacks 28.1% of a New York sample and 25.1% of a national sample sought advice from a friend or family member, 9.7 and 4.0% sought services from a psychologist, counselor, or other therapist, and 11.4 and 11.2% sought advice from a priest, minister, or other religious leader [22].

For many New Yorkers, as well as individuals throughout the country, their emotional reactions to the disaster directly affected their behavior and their outlook on life. Roger Parrino, a Lieutenant in a detective squad in East Harlem, reported to Jim Dwyer of the *New York Times*, "I'm not going to be the same guy…and I'm not going to pretend that life isn't going to be different" [23]. Dwyer further said that, "many who had close encounters with death on Tuesday are finding that not just the skyline has been altered; their own interior landscapes have been rearranged in ways that are still unfolding" [23]. In addition, a study conducted by NORC found that at 4–6 months post September 11, 15.2% of New York residents and 7.6% of a national sample had canceled a plane trip since September 11, 27% of New Yorkers and 16.2% nationally avoided crowded public places, and 5.2% of New Yorkers and 6.7% nationally had reported a suspicious person or activity to the police [22]. Government enforced security measures also changed to account for the uncertainty after September 11, 2001. For example, within a couple of days of the attack, the Federal Aviation Administration prohibited knives of all sizes onboard planes, ended curbside check-in, eliminated cargo and mail from passenger jets, and heightened scrutiny of planes between flights and of unattended vehicles [24].

In addition to the grief, fear, and vulnerability felt by many after the September 11 attacks, within days many also experienced anger and a need to hold someone accountable. Arabs and Muslims within the United States became a target of much of this anger. Somini Sengupta highlighted examples of the rage targeted at innocent

Arabs and Muslims in a *New York Times* article. Sengupta wrote, "on a quiet block in Brooklyn Heights yesterday, a small cluster of men and boys gathered inside a mosque for afternoon prayers." Outside, a man drove past slowly and yelled 'murderers' [25]. Other examples include the windows of a mosque in suburban Dallas being shattered by gunshots, a bag of blood being left outside of a mosque in San Francisco, and bricks thrown through the windows of an Islamic bookstore in Alexandria, VA [25].

Nationally, anger and determination to hold the perpetrators accountable quickly took hold. President Bush and his administration, setting the tone, said that they would "make no distinction between the terrorists who committed these acts and those who harbor them" [26]. Newspapers echoed the growing need to blame and punish with headlines splattered across their pages: "A Somber Bush Says Terrorism Cannot Prevail" [26]; "America Itching for a Fight – War on Terror" [27]; "Vengeful America May Strike at Taliban" [28]; "Terror in America: All Roads Lead to Osama as FBI Unravel Intricate Plot" [29]. By the evening of September 11, 2001 NATO also proclaimed their alliance with the United States, "Our message to the people of the United States is that we are with you. Our message to those who perpetrated these unspeakable crimes is equally clear: you will not get away with it" [30].

As people learned of the loss or survival of friends and family and as the response gained momentum, identification of the vulnerabilities that influenced the events of September 11, 2001 started. One obvious failure in the emergency response to the attacks was the location of New York's crisis center on the 23rd floor of 7 World Trade Center. The command center "was reduced to rubble" [31]. The inadequate disaster preparation within the WTC was publicly recognized, particularly in light of the 1993 attack on the towers. In hindsight, the director of New York Mayor's OEM, Richard Sheirer, recognized the weaknesses in the city's disaster preparedness and stated, "we have learned a lot of lessons and we will make sure that those lessons are put to good use" [31]. Independent committees were established (such as the contracting of McKinsey and Company) to assess the strengths and weaknesses of the response effort and determine the systematic failures or equipment inadequacies that negatively affected the agency's ability to respond effectively (Image 20.3).

The significant loss of response personnel (fire fighters and paramedics) "fueled a quiet reassessment of the first rule of fire rescue: run toward danger when lives are at risk" [32]. In a new era of awareness of the potential of unanticipated disasters, when "suicide hijackers can turn skyscraper steel to spaghetti," Cortez Lawrence, director of national fire programs with the US Fire Administration, a division of the Federal Emergency Management Agency (FEMA), stated that "this is going to require considerable introspection and decisions about who we in the fire service are, and who we're supposed to be" [32]. Los Angeles Battalion Chief Robert Franco suggested that "knowing what we know now, and seeing what we saw at the World Trade Center, in a situation like that you definitely have to consider the possibility of not sending people in" [32]. Arthur Cote of the National Fire Protection Association in Quincy, warned that "there will be a discussion about whether our tactics and our standard procedures are adequate…the only caution is we need not to overreact. Remember this was a very, very unusual situation" [32].

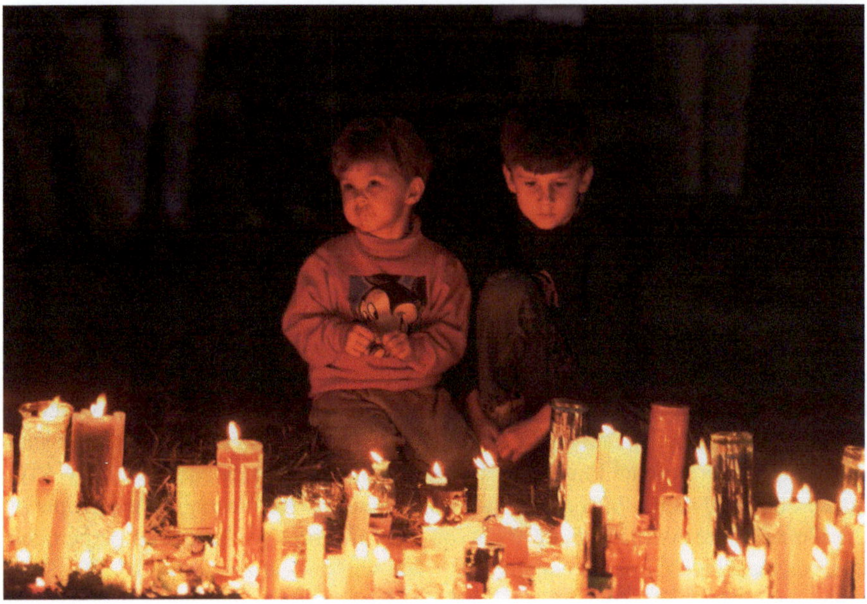

Image 20.3 A vigil in Manhattan following the September 11, 2001 terrorist attacks. Source: Associated Press

Stage Four: Externalizing

In the weeks following the attacks on the United States extensive efforts were made to identify those responsible. By September 26, 2001 one man was arrested and charged with aiding one of the suspected hijackers. Another man was co-operating with law enforcement [27]. John Ashcroft, United States Attorney-General, informed Congress on September 25, 2001 that 352 people had been arrested or detained and that another 392 were wanted for questioning [27]. Mr. Ashcroft further petitioned law-makers to approve legislation that gave law enforcement authorities greater freedoms to combat terrorism. Mr. Ashcroft argued that it is "essential that 'we provide law enforcement with tools necessary to identify, dismantle, disrupt, and punish terrorist organizations before they strike again'" [27].

By September 13, 2001 Osama Bin Laden was targeted as the mastermind of the attacks. Further investigations led the United States government to believe Bin Laden had been given refuge by the Taliban in Afghanistan. Consequently, in an effort to retaliate and destroy the enemy, the United States, with international support, began bomb attacks in Afghanistan on October 7, 2001, just 4 weeks after the terrorist attacks. The bombing targeted Taliban military and communication facilities and suspected terrorist training camps. Eight years later, the United States Military and the military of several international allies, remain in active combat with Afghanistan. Additionally, in the post September 11 context, President Bush and his administration identified another threat, Saddam Hussein's regime in Iraq.

Consequently, with the mission set "to disarm Iraq of weapons of mass destruction, to end Saddam Hussein's support for terrorism, and to free the Iraqi people," on March 20, 2003 President Bush ordered the US military to invade Iraq [33]. Despite the controversy that has since surrounded these two wars, they both clearly represented an attempt to redress perceived vulnerabilities in the US that contributed to the September 11 disaster.

The magnitude of the September 11 terrorist attacks caught all response agencies by surprise and highlighted vulnerabilities within the nation's security measures, disaster preparedness, and response agencies. Immediately following the attacks security along the United States' borders was tightened, security within US embassies throughout the world was enhanced, and travel security guidelines were increased [34]. To evaluate the successes and failings of the United States national security and the local and federal disaster preparedness and response, numerous independent committees were assembled to thoroughly assess the events surrounding September 11, 2001 and to make recommendations on how to improve our safety and emergency services going forward.

In November 2002, the National Commission on Terrorist Attacks Upon the United States was assembled by the United States government to spearhead an all-inclusive review of the events surrounding the September 11, 2001 terrorist attacks on the US. This comprehensive report, the 9-11 Commission Report, presented to President Bush on July 22, 2004, assessed topics such as national security and the emergency response in New York [5].

On a more local level, McKinsey & Company was hired by the Fire Department of New York to critique FDNY and Emergency response efforts and to propose steps for improvement. After 5 months of working with the FDNY, McKinsey & Company published a detailed account of the events of September 11, 2001, focusing specifically on the response efforts of the NYPD, FDNY, and EMS. Pertaining to the FDNY and EMS, the report targeted four categories of weakness: operational preparedness, planning and management, communication and technology capabilities, and system for family and member services [35]. After the release of the report, Mayor Bloomberg announced "the findings of the McKinsey report illustrate both the strengths and weaknesses of the New York Police Department and Fire Department in handling large-scale emergencies, and provide significant opportunities for these vitally important agencies to improve their ability to respond to potential crisis situations in the future" [36]. Many changes followed. Of note, after the release of this report, the New York City Fire Commissioner, Nicholas Scoppetta, announced the creation of the FDNY Terrorism and Disaster Preparedness Strategy, which aimed to "implement a more streamlined, Department-wide approach to emergency response, training, equipment, acquisition and long-term planning" [37]. In addition, in the summer of 2003 Commissioners Scoppetta and Kelly of the FDNY and NYDP, respectively, agreed on a protocol outlining "'unified command'" in the presence of a disaster [38]. This system, which was not in place in 2001, required that in future multi-agency response efforts officials from the NYPD and FDNY work together to coordinate the response effort in the event of a disaster [36, 38] (Image 20.4).

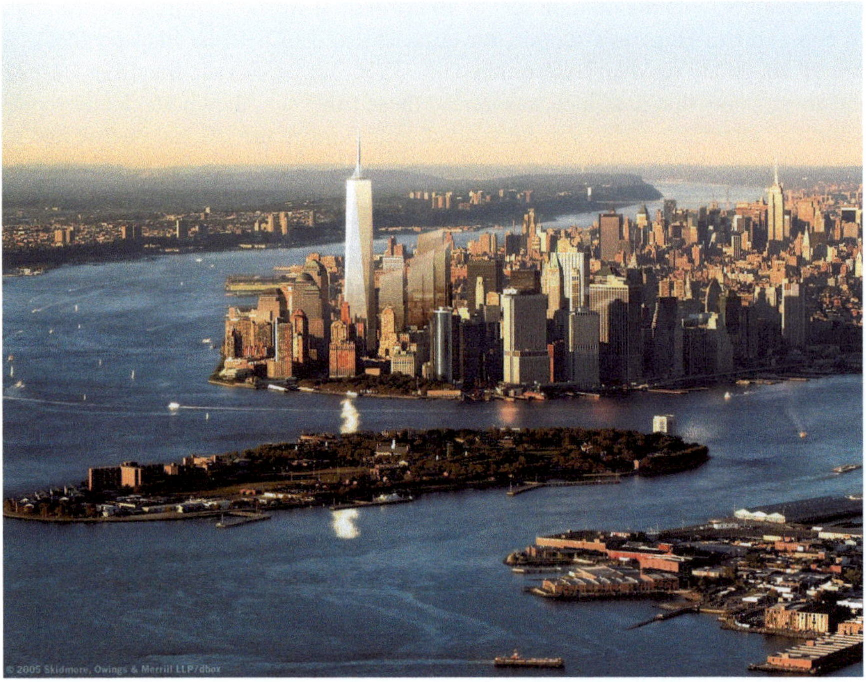

Image 20.4 The Freedom Tower designed to be the first building and memorial to be built at the site of the World Trade Center. Source: Reuters

Stage Five: Renormalization

The September 11, 2001 terrorist attacks on the United States permanently changed the country's sense of vulnerability. In an article assessing "Are New Yorkers Any Safer" 1 year after September 11, 2001, the Gotham Gazette reported the results of a poll conducted by the Daily News showing that 72% of New Yorkers believed another terrorist attack was likely or somewhat likely [39]. Unlike some other countries, such as Israel or Spain, where terrorist attacks have become a tragic but known experience, prior to September 11, 2001 the United States had very little history of large-scale terrorist attacks. However, over the past decade, the attacks have changed the US public's perception of the threats it faces and contributed to substantial changes in population behavior.

For example, scrutiny of aviation security measures for airplane passengers intensified after September 11, 2001. By January 2002, all checked baggage in US commercial airports passed through security to check for explosives. Passengers were restricted from carrying knives, screwdrivers, box cutters, or objects used in cutting on international and domestic flights [40]. In reaction to the continued exposure to terrorist threats, such as Richard Reid – the shoe bomber – airline security procedures have continued to develop. New regulations dictate the amount of liquid each passenger can carry through security as a way of addressing the threat of liquid explosive ingredients. Although these changes may have been unexpected at the time of their introduction, they soon became part of the fabric of everyday life, very much a new, post-disaster, normal.

References

1. Lipton E, Glanz J. Ground zero: firefighting; 9/11 inspires call to review response plan for crises. The New York Times, B 4. January 23, 2002.
2. McPhee M, Saltonstall D, Colangelo LL. What went wrong on 9/11 two reports detail FDNY, NYPD woes. Daily News. August 20, 2002:News,10.
3. New York City Department of Health. 9/11 Health: historical context. http://www.nyc.gov/html/doh/wtc/html/background/background.shtml. Accessed 20 Sept 2009.
4. National Commission of Terrorist Attacks Upon the United States. The 9/11 commission report: executive summary. Washington, DC: United States Government; 2004;Executive summary. http://www.gpoaccess.gov/911/pdf/execsummary.pdf. Accessed June 2009.
5. National Commission on Terrorist Attacks. The 9/11 commission report. Government Printing Office; 2004:1–585. http://govinfo.library.unt.edu/911/report/index.htm. Accessed June 2009.
6. National Commission on Terrorist Attacks. The 9/11 commission report. Government Printing Office; 2004:293. http://govinfo.library.unt.edu/911/report/index.htm. Accessed June 2009.
7. Averill JD, Mileti DS, Peacock RD, et al. Federal building and fire safety investigation of the World Trade Center disasters. Occupant behavior, egress, and emergency communications. Washington, DC: U.S. Government Printing Office; 2005;NIST NCSTAR 1–7:1–298. http://wtc.nist.gov/NCSTAR1/PDF/NCSTAR%201-7.pdf. Accessed June 2009.
8. Walsh MW. At 8:48 a.m., two 'normal guys' met a moment of transformation. The New York Times, A 16. September 16, 2001.
9. National Commission on Terrorist Attacks. The 9/11 commission report. Government Printing Office; 2004:299. http://govinfo.library.unt.edu/911/report/index.htm. Accessed June 2009.
10. Kleinfield NR. A creeping horror: buildings burn and fall as onlookers search for elusive safety. The New York Times. September 12, 2001;August 29, 2007 Press Release #076-07:1.
11. Purnick J. Metro matters; city turns, temporarily, into a small town. The New York Times, A 6. September 12, 2001.
12. Ojito M. After the attacks: the volunteers; lending everything from ears to elbow grease. The New York Times, A 11. September 13, 2001.
13. Kennedy R. A day of terror: transportation; with city transit shut down, New Yorkers take to eerily empty streets. The New York Times, A 8. September 12, 2001.
14. South Africans traumatised by Tuesday's US drama. South African Press Association. September 12, 2001.
15. Harmon A. A day of terror: the talk online; web offers both news and comfort. The New York Times, A 25. September 12, 2001.
16. ShunnB."I'mOkRegistry".http://webarchives.loc.gov/collections/lcwa0001/20020913002326/http://www.shunn.net/okay/. Accessed 6 June 2009.
17. James C. A day of terror: critic's notebook; live images make viewers witnesses to horror. The New York Times, A 25. September 12, 2001.
18. Wetzstein C. Poll: nation depressed about terror. The Washington Times. September 20, 2001:Nation,A 8.
19. Appleby J, Armour S. USA begins to deal with grief over attacks. USA Today. September 20, 2001:Money,1 B.
20. Galea S, Resnick H, Ahern J, et al. Posttraumatic stress disorder in Manhattan, New York City, after the September 11th terrorist attacks. J Urban Health. 2002;79:340–53.

21. One in eight WTC rescue and recovery workers developed post-traumatic stress disorder. New findings from the World Trade Center health registry show rates were highest among volunteer workers, lowest among police officers. New York: New York City Department of Health and Mental Hygiene; 2007;August 29 2007 Press Release #076-07. http://www.nyc.gov/html/doh/html/pr2007/pr076-07.shtml. Accessed June 2009.
22. Rasinski KA, Berktold J, Smith TW, Albertson BL. America recovers: a follow-up to a national study of public responses to the September 11th terrorist attacks. Chicago, IL: A National Organization for Research, University of Chicago; August 7 2002. http://www.norc.uchicago.edu/NR/rdonlyres/E80028D8-96BB-47EF-90A3-B69D253D8652/0/pubresp2.pdf. Accessed June 2006.
23. Dwyer J. After the attacks: close calls; survivors who barely made it out in time try to cope with grim fact that others did not. The New York Times, A 9. September 14, 2001.
24. McFadden RD. After the attacks: the overview; stunned rescuers comb attack sites, but thousands are presumed dead; F.B.I. tracking hijackers' movements. The New York Times, A 1. September 13, 2001.
25. Sengupta S. Arabs and muslims steer through an unsettling scrutiny. The New York Times, A 24. September 13, 2001.
26. Bumiller E, Sanger DE. A day of terror: The President; a somber Bush says terrorism cannot revail. The New York Times, A 1. September 12, 2001.
27. Eccleston R. American public itching for a fight – war on terror. The Australian. September 26, 2001:World,13.
28. Masanauskas J. Vengeful US may strike at Taliban. Herald Sun. September 13, 2001:News,11.
29. Terror in America: all roads lead to Osama as FBI unravel intricate plot. Birmingham Post. September 14, 2001:4.
30. NATO promises "assistance and support" for U.S. Deutsche Presse-Agentur (International News). September 11, 2001.
31. Baker A, Flynn K. Once, it was a monument to preparedness; officials seek best location, and a backup, for a new command center. The New York Times, D 1. September 29, 2001.
32. Zuckoff M. America prepares/the investigation; firefighters reassess policy of rushing in. The Boston Globe. September 26, 2001:National/Foreign,A1.
33. Bush GW. President discusses beginning of operation Iraqi freedom. Washington, DC: The White House, Office of the Press Secretary; 2003;President's Radio Address. http://georgewbush-whitehouse.archives.gov/news/releases/2003/03/20030322.html. Accessed 6 June 2009.
34. Gardiner B. World Watches in horror as terror unfolds in New York. The Daily Record, A 9. September 11, 2001. http://news.google.com/newspapers?nid=860&dat=20010911&id=hywfAAAAIBAJ&sjid=jccEAAAAIBAJ&pg=1269,1687837. Accessed 6 June 2009.
35. McKinsey & Company. McKinsey report – increasing FDNY's preparedness. McKinsey & Company; 2002. http://www.nyc.gov/html/fdny/html/mck_report/toc.html. Accessed 20 June 2009.
36. Smith S. McKinsey report examines NYC response to 9/11. http://ehstoday.com/news/ehs_imp_35764/. Accessed 6 June 2009.
37. Scoppetta N. FDNY releases terrorism and disaster preparedness strategy. http://www.nyc.gov/html/fdny/html/events/2007/042507a.shtml. Accessed 6 June 2009.
38. Rashbaum WK, O'Donnell M. City police and fire department pledge cooperation in disasters. The New York Times, A 1. July 12, 2003.
39. Vitullo-Martin J. 9/11/01-02: are New Yorkers any safer. http://www.gothamgazette.com/crime/91102.shtml. Accessed 6 June 2009.
40. McClure G. Has airport security improved since 9/11? http://www.todaysengineer.org/2005/Jun/security.asp. Accessed 6 June 2009.

Chapter 21
Disasters from a Public Health Perspective

How Can We Use the Models?

Throughout this book we have offered two models. Grounding our thinking in the rich literature that over the past few decades has refined our conceptualization of disasters; we used a unique database both to inform the models and to provide evidence that each of the models is consistent with on-the-ground realities. The models are by design flexible enough to accommodate the heterogeneity of hazards, vulnerabilities, and behaviors observed in a range of disaster experiences. It is our intention that the two models proposed might be useful to frame how we think about population health interventions that target the proximate and long-term causes and consequences of disasters.

Our model of the formation of disasters is based on the notion that disasters are not unexpected externally imposed events. Instead, we posit that they are created through an interaction between the hazard and underlying context. This renders disaster mitigation a top priority; disaster outcomes cannot be dismissed as unavoidable natural events. Therefore, the onus of averting the consequences of disasters falls back on us. Accepting this, disaster mitigation efforts may do well to shift attention away from hazards to underlying conditions of the hazard-affected areas. The focus on singular hazards, or even types of hazards, may be futile in the absence of a clear understanding of the pre-existing structural and institutional factors that allow a disaster to occur.

Our model of population behavior, which is predicated on the literature and the case studies in our dataset, suggests a predictability of human responses to disasters. We can expect behaviors during and after disasters to conform to a set sequence and we expect that these behaviors will, for the most part, be rational. The understanding that behavioral responses to disasters are both predictable and rational introduces an opportunity to promote life-saving, damage-minimizing behaviors following disasters. In addition, it suggests the scope of potential institutional interventions that could address expected population needs in the aftermath of these events.

S. Rudenstine and S. Galea, *The Causes and Behavioral Consequences of Disasters: Models Informed by the Global Experience* 1950–2005, DOI 10.1007/978-1-4614-0317-3_21, © Springer Science+Business Media, LLC 2012

In presenting both these models in a single book, we sought to bridge the conversation regarding how disasters form, on one hand, and what happens after disasters, on the other. While the models are distinct, they operate in concert with one another. That is, the combination of factors that produce the disaster affects how the population responds to the disaster, and conversely, population behavior after a disaster influences underlying vulnerabilities and capacities that will interact with future hazards.

Pragmatically, continuity between the pre- and post-disaster period is critical. The first model describes how an existing environment, characterized by vulnerabilities and capacities, may become disturbed by an external hazard. Subsequently, additional stressors or protectors that are incidental to the hazard itself may modify the effects of this interaction. The model of population behavior begins where the first model ends – the disaster itself. New population behaviors emerge to accommodate disaster circumstances. For example, internalizing, stage three of the behavior model, describes the group search for whom or what to blame. The sequence of blame mirrors the major factors involved in disaster evolution. Externalizing, stage four, begins with identifying the hazard itself (e.g., the terrorist attack or a hurricane), and then focuses on the intermittent stressors that aggravated negative outcomes. In renormalization, stage five, the population recognizes and accepts the role of underlying vulnerabilities in determining the magnitude of disaster.

For example, during the New York City Subway Fire in 1990, described in Chap. 8, the communication system proved inadequate in the context of the hazard, leading to delayed rescue [1]. However, an error in the electrical wiring of the subway tracks was the underlying cause of the fire [2]. Initial public response to the disaster was blame and anger aimed at those responsible for laying the original electrical wiring of the Subway system. As details of the disaster were made known, public blame shifted to the Transit Authority for communication failures and poor maintenance of the subway tunnel, both of which enhanced the disaster. The corrections made to the subway system, such as increased subway track maintenance following this disaster were directly influenced by public perception that negligence was a large contributor to the disaster's formation.

It is worth noting that externalizing behaviors, largely taking place in stage four, essentially modify the underlying regional conditions that will become important in the context of future hazards. Externalizing is contingent on culprits (human and systemic) identified during the internalizing stage, and is the process through which perceived vulnerabilities are rectified. During the normalizing stage, in stage five, new behaviors that were originally enacted in response to the disaster become the standard societal norm. Externalizing and normalizing together set the stage for the hazards that will subsequently occur, clearly linking both models over time.

Implications of the Models for Public Health

The population health consequences of disasters are broad and can include in the short- and long-term increases in rates of injury, psychopathology, infectious diseases, and mortality among those affected by the event. These direct health consequences are compounded by the indirect health effects of destroyed public infrastructure and lost individual assets that in many cases may have more marked and longer-term consequences than the direct effects.

Although disasters are episodic, we suggest that our understanding of disasters benefits from the systematic study of disasters as a whole. An approach that is limited to isolated inquiry about individual events will fall short of capturing the full range of consequences after disaster events or the patterns of determinants that shape these consequences. Health consequences, just as disasters themselves, are not inevitable. To the contrary, they will depend on the type of hazard, the level of institutional preparedness, and degree of vulnerability to the stressors produced during the disaster, to name a few. Moreover, the health burden of disasters is not randomly distributed. To a large extent, the distribution of hazard exposure and disaster consequences among the population (i.e., who will be affected) is determined by the factors introduced in the model on *the causes of* disasters – specifically, systemic characteristics predating the hazard which would be only marginally changed by the post-disaster response. This resonates with the popular observation that areas are vulnerable to specific types of hazards, and hence the common use of "earthquake-prone" or "flood-prone" to describe areas. We know that vulnerabilities are associated with particular areas, which then in turn affect the population's risk of disaster. Moreover, we have argued that hazards and vulnerabilities are interdependent, and that vulnerability to a hazard and susceptibility to disaster damages overlap. This implies an urgency to intervene on these characteristics. Household poverty, for example, forces people to reside in unsafe areas – whether areas prone to natural hazards such as low lying flood plains, areas near industrial sites, or crowded inner cities without infrastructural amenities. Household poverty also makes individuals more susceptible to negative health outcomes arising from the disaster. Because communities that are more likely to experience hazards are less able to cope with them, any improvement in the underlying conditions may have a doubly powerful effect on disaster consequences.

Torrential rains in several Colombian regions in May 2005 caused flooding and mudslides in those communities near rivers and mountains. Poor architectural design and construction of homes contributed to the disaster and outcomes. For example, many people dismissed construction guidelines regarding proper drainage systems, leaving their homes vulnerable to flooding in heavy rains [3]. Another example occurred during heavy and long-lasting storms throughout the US west coast in February 1986. After days of strong winds and rain a "crumbling levee in northern California" collapsed leading to the additional evacuation of 21,000 residents of the area [4]. Response teams worked quickly to fill in the levee with rocks and dirt, but the devastation from the initial break was irreversible [4, 5].

Building on our model of the causes of disasters, we argue that multiple layers of the social, political, and economic contexts are inextricably linked to the production of disasters. Thus effective interventions must consider each level (e.g., household, neighborhood, region) and domain of influence (e.g., governance, geography, culture). This again underscores the importance for multidisciplinary inquiry and action in the disaster context – any single approach is likely to be too narrow to capture the full complexity of the relevant determinants. While individual level factors are important for recovery from disasters, individuals generally do not have the ability to prevent the disaster event itself. Rather, it is public institutions and officials who might have the power to modify the structural environment to thwart disasters. This suggests that the scope of public health practice in the context of disaster prevention and mitigation needs to be broadened to include attention to structural features shaping population vulnerability to disasters. It may then be argued that social, political, and economic policies are all within the domain of public health, and that all policy makers ought to incorporate population health implications into the decision-making process.

The role of the institutional response during disasters is not trivial. Disaster response and recovery planning may be framed around the model of population behavior. The post-disaster behavior model suggests that accurate information is a primary driving factor in rational population behavior. This stresses the importance of transparency throughout the evolution of disasters. As hazards unfold, populations will behave rationally if they are privy to accurate information. For example, in response to the news of Hurricane Lili's movements toward Cuba in October 1996, President Fidel Castro appeared on state television to warn Cubans to prepare for something "catastrophic" [6]. In response to this broadcasting, and other forms of information-seeking behaviors, at least 80,000 people evacuated dangerous dwellings and sought shelter [6].

Additionally, because perceived culpability motivates action during the externalizing stage, it is important for public officials and all those who possess relevant information to actively disseminate it. The confluence of incidental failures should be distinguished from systemic failures openly and honestly. Here, the role of the media is also crucial. The media are in a unique position to inform the general population during disasters as well as to set the tone for action through the type of news broadcasted and the representation of facts. Public health practitioners must acknowledge the important role they play as liaisons with the media and in providing media outlets with timely and accurate reports on disasters. Similarly, our model of population behavior builds on the notion that population responses are predictable, and thus institutional intervention after disasters may be molded to anticipate the expected emerging behaviors. Creating an institutional environment that is attentive to the underlying vulnerabilities and capacities that intersect with hazards to produce disasters will minimize the consequences of disasters. Further, tending to the developing needs of a community after experiencing a disaster could establish an environment that can successfully mitigate the negative health outcomes of disasters.

Conclusion

Building on perspectives from different disciplines, in particular epidemiology, anthropology, sociology, we aimed to present two models, one describing the causes of disasters and other describing the patterns of population behavior after disasters.

We had two central goals in presenting these models. First, we intended this work to be useful to public health thinking and practice. It was our aim to synthesize our thinking about the cause of disasters as well as about the patterns of population behavior after these events in a way that was accessible and useful to those who were in a position to intervene both on the factors that may cause disasters and on the drivers of population behavior in their aftermath. Second, we hoped to contribute to the body of scholarly work about disasters. Although, as we have recognized throughout this book, there is a large and growing body of work that has considered how disasters are caused, there is much less work that has explicitly offered models of population behavior after these events. Our aim here then was to help clarify work about the cause of disasters, and to advance the field in thinking about population behaviors after these events. We hope that we have achieved some of that goal, and even more importantly, that our work will encourage others to tackle the issues presented here in a way that further informs practice and scholarship in the area.

References

1. Beckman EB, Pers I, Davitt K, Turkewitz B, Banks J. An analysis of the agency response to The December 28, 1990 smoke and fire condition at the Clark Street Station. New York City: The Council of the City of New York; 1991.
2. Sims C. Subway agency blames old error for fatal fire. The New York Times. 1991:23.
3. In Colombia 16 dead, 30 injured in torrential rains. Agence France-Presse. 2005.
4. Associated Press. California levee crumbles; 21,000 more evacuated. The Washington Post. 1986:A,3.
5. Thousands crowd shelter in flood. The New York Times. 1986:1.
6. Hurricane Lili Hits Cuba. http://www.cnn.com/WEATHER/9610/18/lili. Accessed 8 Nov 2006.

Index

S. Rudenstine and S. Galea, *The Causes and Behavioral Consequences of Disasters: Models Informed by the Global Experience* 1950–2005,
DOI 10.1007/978-1-4614-0317-3, © Springer Science+Business Media, LLC 2012

MIX
Papier aus verantwortungsvollen Quellen
Paper from responsible sources
FSC® C105338

If you have any concerns about our products,
you can contact us on
ProductSafety@springernature.com

In case Publisher is established outside the EU,
the EU authorized representative is:
Springer Nature Customer Service Center GmbH
Europaplatz 3, 69115 Heidelberg, Germany

Printed by Libri Plureos GmbH
in Hamburg, Germany